W0269320

Anaesthesiology and Resuscitation

Anaesthesiologie und Wiederbelebung

Anesthésiologie et Réanimation

8

Editores

Prof. Dr. R. Frey, Mainz · Dr. F. Kern, St. Gallen
Prof. Dr. O. Mayrhofer, Wien

Third World Congress
of Anaesthesiology

São Paulo, Brazil · September 1964

Panel Discussions

Edited by

P. R. Bromage, J. E. Eckenhoff, R. Frey,
T. Cecil Gray, M. Digby Leigh,
Sir Robert R. Macintosh, L. E. Morris, J. A. Nesi,
C. R. Ritsema van Eck, M. Zindler

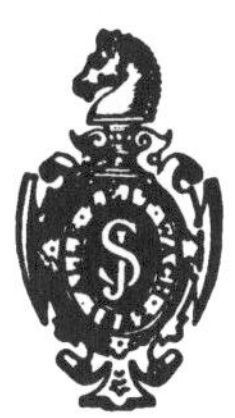

Springer-Verlag Berlin Heidelberg GmbH 1966

ISBN 978-3-662-23209-5   ISBN 978-3-662-25215-4 (eBook)
DOI 10.1007/978-3-662-25215-4

Library of Congress Catalog Card Number 66-25390

Preface

The official papers of the Third World Congress of Anaesthesiology appeared during the Congress at São Paulo 1964. All participants appreciated highly the immense editorial work done by the Congress President Dr. Rodriges Alves and the Secretary, Doctor Carlos Parsloe, Hospital Samaritano, São Paulo, Brazil.

The 10 panels of the World Congress created much interest. Not only the scientific committee, but also many anaesthesiologists all over the world requested that a report of these discussions on remarkable points of interest be made available.

The editors of "Anaesthesiology and Resuscitation" therefore collected all material available. They want to thank all chairmen and members of the panels for their help and advice, Doctor Carlos Parsloe from São Paulo and his colleagues of the Committee for the Third World Congress at São Paulo for their valuable assistance, and last not least their publisher for his untiring cooperation.

Mainz, 1966   RUDOLF FREY

Contents

Participants

AMARAL, R. V. G., M. D., São Paulo, Brazil

ARTUSIO, J. F., M. D., Anaesthesiologist-in-Chief, The New York Hospital – Cornell Medical Center, New York, U.S.A.

BEARD, J., M. D., F.F.A.R.C.S., Department of Anaesthetics, Hammersmith and National Heart Hospital, London, England

BIANHCETTI, L., M. D. (in absence of E. CIOCATTO, M. D., Professor of Anaesthesiology, University of Turin)

BROMAGE, P. R., M. B., B. S., F.F.A.R.C.S., Assistant Professor of Anaesthesia, McGill University and Royal Victoria Hospital, Montreal, Canada

BROWN, A. S., M. B., Ch. B., F.F.A.R.C.S., Edinburgh, England

CIOCATTO, E., M. D., Professor of Anaesthesiology, University of Turin, Italy

CONN, A. W., M. D., F.R.C.P. (C.), Anaesthetist-in-Chief, The Hospital for Sick Children, Toronto, Canada

CORSSEN, G., M. D., Professor of Anaesthesiology, University Hospital, Ann Arbor, Michigan, U.S.A.

CRUL, J. F., M. D., Professor of Anaesthesiolgy, University of Nijmegen, Netherlands

DOENICKE, A., M. D., Ass. Professor of Anaesthesiology, Head Department of Anaesthesia, Chirurgische Poliklinik University of Munich, Germany

DUNDEE, J. W., M. B., B. Ch., F.F.A.R.C.S. Professor of Anaesthesia, Queen's University of Belfast, Northern Irland

RITSEMA VAN ECK, C. R., M. D., Professor of Anaesthesiology, University of Groningen, Netherlands

ECKENHOFF, J. E., M.D., Professor of Anaesthesiology, University of Pennsylvania, Philadelphia, U.S.A.

ELLIS, S., M. D., Philadelphia, U.S.A.

ENDERBY, G. E. H., M. A., M.B., B.Ch., F.F.A.R.C.S., London, England

ERIKSSON, E. K., M. D., Upplands-Väsvy, Sweden

DE FREITAS L., BRANDAO, M. D., Professor of Anaesthesiology, Falculdade de Medicina de Porto Alegre, Brazil

FREY, R., M. D., F.F.A.R.C.S Professor of Anaesthesiology, University of Mainz, Germany

GAUTHIER-LAFAY, P. J., M. D., Departement d'Anesthésiologie, Université de Strassbourg, France

GEDDES, I. C., M. D., F.F.A.R.C.S., Department of Anaesthesia, University of Liverpool, England

GEMPERLE, M., M. D., Head of the Department of Anaesthesia, University of Geneva, Geneva, Switzerland

GHOSE, R., M. D., Addis Abeba, Africa

GOLDMAN, V., M.R.C.S., L.R.C.P., F.F.A.R.C.S., London, England

GOMEZ, Q. J., M. D., Manila, Philipines

GORDON, R. A., M. D., Toronto, Canada

GRAY, T. C., M. D., F.F.A.R.C.S., Professor of Anaesthesia, University of Liverpool, England

GREENE, N. M., M. D., Professor of Anaesthesiology, Yale University, New Haven, Connecticut

HAMILTON, W. K., M. D., Department of Anaesthesiology, University of Iowa, Iowa City, U.S.A.

HENSCHEL, W. F., M. D., Head of the Department of Anaesthesia, Städtische Krankenanstalten, Bremen, Germany

HINGSON, R. A., M. D., L.L.D., D.H.L., Professor of Anaesthesia, Western Reserve University, Cleveland, Ohio, U.S.A.

HOLMDAHL, M. H., M. D., Professor of Anaesthesiology, Akademiska Sjukhuset, Uppsala, Sweden

HOWELLS, T., D. A., F.F.A.R.C.S., Royal Free Hospital, London, England

ILLES, I. A., M. D., Illinois Masonic Hospital, Chicago, Illinois, U.S.A.

IWAI, S., M. D., Head, Department of Anaesthesiology, National Children's Hospital, Tokyo, Japan

IWATSUKI, K., M. D., Professor of Anaesthesiology, Tohoku University School of Medicine, Sendai, Japan

JOHNSTONE, M. W., M. B., B. Ch., F.F.A.R.C.S., The University of Manchester, The Royal Infirmary, Manchester, England

KEERI–SZANTO, M., M. D., Montreal, Canada

KOK, O.V.S., M. D., Professor of Anaesthesiology, University of Pretoria, South Africa

KUCHER, R., M. D., Ass. Professor of Anaesthesiology, University of Vienna, Austria

LARENG, L., M. D., Professeur d'Anesthésiologie, Université de Toulouse, France

LEIGH, M. Digby, M. D., Head, Division of Anaesthesiology, Children's Hospital of Los Angeles, California, U.S.A.

LEWIS, G. B., jr., M. D., Children's Hospital of Los Angeles, U.S.A.

Sir MACINTOSH, Robert R., D. M., F.R.C.S., F.F.A.R.C.S., Nuffield Professor of Anaesthetics, Oxford, England

MORRIS, L. E., M. D., Director, Anaesthesia Research Laboratories, Providence Hospital, (and) Clinical Professor, University of Washington, Seattle, U.S.A.

MUSHIN, W. W., M. A., M. B., B. S., F.F.A.R.C.S., Professor of Anaesthetics, Welsh National School of Medicine, University of Wales, Cardiff, U. K.

NESI, J. A., M. D., Professor of Anaesthesiology, University of Caracas, Venezuela

NILSSON, E., M. D., Professor of Anaesthesiology, Lasarettet, Lund, Sweden

ODURO, K. A., M. D., Accra, Ghana/Africa

OECH, St. R., M. D., Department of Anaesthesiology, Lankenau Hospital, Philadelphia, Pennsylvania, U.S.A.

ORGANE, G. S. W., M. D., F.F.A.R.C.S., Professor of Anaesthesia, Westminster Hospital, London, England

PAYNE, J. P., M. B., Ch. B., F.F.A.R.C.S., Professor of Anaesthesia, Hammersmith Hospital, London, England

POULSEN, H., M. D., Professor of Anaesthesiology, University of Aarhus, Denmark

REES, G. J., M. B., Ch. B., F.F.A.R.C.S., Department of Anaesthesia, The University of Liverpool, England

Radnay, P. A., M. D., Rockland State Hospital, New York, U.S.A.

Sankawa, H., M. D., Division of Anaesthesiology. Children's Hospital, Los Angeles, U.S.A.

Sellick, B. A., M. B., B. S., F.F.A.R.C.S., London, England

Smith, R. M., M. D., The Children's Hospital Medical Center, Boston, Mass., U.S.A.

Stead, A. L., M. B., Ch. B., F.F.A.R.C.S., Liverpool, England

Stephens, K. F., O. B. E., M. B., B. S., F.F.A.R.C.S., London, England

Truant, A. P., Ph. D., Laboratory of Biological Research, Astra Pharmaceutical Products, Inc., Worcester, Mass., U.S.A.

Usubiaga, J. E., M. D., Hospital Rivadavia, Buenos Aires, Argentina. (Present address: Jackson Memorial Hospital, Miami, Florida, U.S.A.)

Wakai, I., M. D., Nagoya, Japan

Wolfe, L., M. D., Ph. D., Chief of Neurochemistry, McGill University and Montreal Neurological Institute, Montreal, Canada

Yamamura, H., M. D., Professor of Anaesthesiology, Tokyo University Hospital, Bunkyo-ko, Tokyo, Japan

Zindler, M., M. D., Professor of Anaesthesiology, University of Düsseldorf, Germany

Introduction to the panel on catecholamines and their significance in anaesthesia

R. Frey

For many years catecholamines and sympathomimetic drugs have been used to combat certain types of cardiac depression and hypotension. The development of very sensitive methods for the determination of catecholamine levels in urine, plasma and tissue now allows us to study the normal response of the body to different anaesthetics and to the challenges of surgical trauma. Many new drugs employed in the treatment of arterial hypertension profoundly affect the sympathetic nervous system by many mechanisms and we, therefore, meet in our hypertensive patients new and difficult problems during anaesthesia and postoperatively. In addition to all this, drugs like epinephrine have strong metabolic effects. Thus, there are many old and new reasons for a discussion of catecholamines in anaesthesia.

Panel Discussions on

A. Catecholamines and their significance in anaesthesia

Chairman: R. Frey, Mainz
Members: J. Beard, London; P. J. Gauthier-Lafay, Villeneuve-Sur-Lot;
N. M. Greene, New Haven; R. Kucher, Vienna; L. Lareng, Toulouse;
St. R. Oech, Philadelphia.

I. Principles and observations

a) Opening of the panel

Chairman: The adrenergic (ergotropic) responses of the body to psychological and/or physiological stress ("aggression") are influenced not only by the Nervous System, but also *humoral* factors: The HORMONES.

They are absolutely necessary for fight or flight and intensive studies are mandatory in the future.

The object of our panel is:

To show the problem,

to ask questions and to be critical of the dogmas of the past!

First a word on nomenclature:

The main subjects of our discussion will be the two hormones of the adrenal gland:

Adrenalin (Epinephrie) and

Nor-Adrenalin (Nor-Epinephrie).

Under physiological conditions these two substances never occur alone but always together.

b) Basic anatomy and physiology of the sympathetic nervous system

N. M. Greene

Anatomically the sympathetic nervous system is comprised of central and peripheral portions. The central or medullary portions of the sympathetic nervous system are adjacent to the respiratory center. As recently demonstrated by PRICE, there are several functionally different areas of the sympathetic nervous system at this level and, for example, an agent such as cyclopropane apparently increases total sympathetic outflow by depressing the inhibitory center of the central portion of the sympathetic nervous system (H. L. PRICE, et al., Anaesthesiology **24**: 1, 1963).

Peripherally, the sympathetic nervous system consists of the wellknown pre- and post-ganglionic arrangement of fibers. From an anaesthetic point of view two things deserve emphasis. First, in conduction anaesthetic technics such as spinal anaesthesia wherein preganglionic sympathetic block is produced, sympathetic denervation will be complete when the preganglionic fibers at T1 are blocked. Because sympathetic fibers are blocked, on the average, 2 spinal segments above the level made sensory to pinprick during spinal anaesthesia (GREENE, Anaesthesiology **19**: 45, 1958), when sensory anaesthesia extends to T3, sympathetic denervation is complete. As a corollary, sympathetic block is no greater with cervical levels of spinal anaesthesia than with high thoracic levels. Accordingly, since the vascular response to spinal anaesthesia is mediated only through the sympathetics, the vascular response to spinal anaesthesia is no greater with cervical levels than with high Thoracic levels.

Secondly, each preganglionic fiber ascends and descends in the paravertebral sympathetic chain where it anastamoses with up to 22 postganglionic fibers. This means that stimulation or (as with spinal) paralysis of a single preganglionic fiber produces a diffuse peripheral response, one that is not segmentally related to the spinal segment at which the preganglionic block occurred.

Finally, it should be borne in mind that postganglionic fibers have as the chemical mediator between themselves and their effector organs norepinephrine. Only the preganglionic sympathetic fibers going to the adrenal medulla cause the release of epinephrine. In this regard increased blood levels of catecholamines as during certain types of anaesthesia are the result of increased sympathetic activity, not the cause of increased sympathetic activity as is so often mistakenly assumed. The increased blood levels of catecholamines associated with increased sympathetic activity may add to the response of effector organs after being hematogenously carried to the effector organs, but the blood levels by themselves are not the primary cause of increased activity.

c) Metabolic effects of catecholamines

N. M. Greene

The most important naturally occurring catecholamines are epinephrine and norepinephrine. They may have metabolic effects because of their direct actions, or because of their indirect effects, or (as is usually the case) by a combination of direct and indirect effects. Norepinephrine has no significant direct effects on metabolism. Epinephrine does, however. The chief direct metabolic effects of epinephrine are exerted on liver and on fat. In the liver, epinephrine stimulates generation of adenosine monophosphate (AMP), a co-factor influencing phosphorylase activity. Phosphorylase is the enzyme responsible for the breakdown of glycogen to glucose-1-phosphate and hence to glucose, but phosphorylase activity is controlled by many factors, including as mentioned, adenosine monphosphate which in turn is influenced by epinephrine. In this regard, it should be remembered that stimulation of the sympathetic nerves going to the liver results in glycolysis and hence in hyperglycemia independently of any simultaneous effect on blood epinephrine levels. Such a hyperglycemia is solely due to the effect of the sympathetic nerves on their effector organs, the hepatic cells themselves. However, if the sympathetic nerve stimulation is widespread enough to involve not only the hepatic sympathetics but also the sympathetic fibers going to the adrenal medulla, then there will also be an increased blood level of epinephrine. The epinephrine will be hematogenously borne to the liver and will increase further the glycolysis and so have an additive effect on the hyperglycemia. It is a mistake to assume that the hyperglycemia of, for example, ether anaesthesia is due solely to the increased blood levels of epinephrine which may be observed in certain species. Such hyperpinephrinemia hematogenously contributes to, but is not the sole cause of, hepatic glycolysis. As a corollary, any anaesthetic which produces increased sympathetic activity will be associated with hyperglycemia. Cyclopropane, for example, is accompanied by a hyperglycemia of approximately the same extent as that associated with ether anaesthesia, a fact not widely reported and not so widely appreciated, and also a fact leading to the amusing and inconsistent statement that ether should not be given to diabetics (because it produces hyperglycemia) while cyclopropane may be given to such patients.

Presumably epinephrine has the same metabolic effect on the glycogen in striated (i. e. skeletal) muscle as it does in liver, though this has not been as widely studied nor is it probably as of great importance from the overall biochemical point of view as is the effect of epinephrine on hepatic glycogen. But the effect of epinephrine on fat metabolism, including glycolysis in fat, probably is as important if not more important than the effect on the liver. Only recently has the metabolic importance of fatty tissue been emphasized and more and more studies are being devoted to this previously underestimated determinant of metabolic response. In future years I predict that the metabolic importance of fatty tissue will become increasingly important, especially in the anaesthetized patient.

But catecholamines, both epinephrine and norepinephrine may also have indirect effects on metabolism by producing changes in tissue oxygenation, that is tissue oxygen tension. They may do this by changing tissue blood flow by producing changes in cardiac output or the degree of peripheral arteriolar vasoconstriction, or they may do this by changing the rate of tissue oxygen consumption (the calorigenic effect of epinephrine), or they may change tissue oxygen tension by a combination of both methods. For example, epinephrine administration is associated with a hyperglycemia and increased blood levels of lactic acid and pyruvic acid which are purely secondary to the increased metabolism. But, in addition epinephrine produces an increase in lactic acid (excess lactate) above and beyond that which can be ascribed to concurrent changes in pyruvic acid. This excess lactate is best explained on the basis of regional areas of anaerobiosis produced by the epinephrine (Greene, J. Lab. Clin. Med. **58**: 682, 1961).

Finally, the indirect metabolic effects of catecholamines are demonstrated in the role they play during anoxic anoxia. Anoxic anoxia is normally accompanied by both a hyperglycemia as well as increased blood lactate and pyruvate levels and the appearance of excess lactate. But such anoxia also strongly stimulates the sympathetic nervous system, and the question arises as to what per cent of the total metabolic response to anoxia may be ascribed to the anoxia per se and what per cent is ascribable to the reflex release of catecholamines produced by the anoxia. Experimental studies in dogs made hypoxic in the presence and absence of an intact sympathetic nervous system (Greene & Phillips, Amer. J. Physiol. **180**: 475, 1957) have shown that approximately 40% of the metabolic response to hypoxia is due to the concurrent release of catecholamines and not to the hypoxia itself. This is but one of the many examples of the indirect effects of catecholamines on metabolism.

d) Changes in catecholamine levels in response to premedication, anaesthesia and surgery

R. Frey and F. W. Ahnefeld *

Plasma catecholamine levels were measured during surgery and anaesthesia with different narcotic agents. In this context a preliminary result is of clinical interest: During Halothane anaesthesia there was sufficient peripheral circulation and moderately lowered blood pressure in spite of increased adrenalin and noradrenalin values. Arterial blood pressure returned to normal $^1/_2$ to 1 hour after completion of anaesthesia. Poor peripheral circulation was now noted in some cases. In these patients it was possible to demonstrate an increase of plasma catecholamine levels in comparison to those found during anaesthesia. The circulating volume showed deficits from 700 to 1300 ml (34 patients). It was possible to stabilize the circulation and normalize the peripheral perfusion by appropriate supply of liquids and sympathicolytic medication.

The findings allow the following interpretation:

1. The effect of catecholamines is diminished during Halothane anaesthesia and a possibly present volume deficit is hardly evident.

2. Vasoconstrictive influence of the catecholamines is increased after cessation of the specific action of Halothane.

Additionally, we observe an increased output of catecholamines probably consequent to hypovolemia.

Adrenalin and noradrenalin normalize blood pressure but reduce the peripheral perfusion at the same time.

Inadequate volume substitution and influence of catecholamines are responsible for the fact that some patients look pale and have collapsed veins in the immediate postoperative period.

In such cases we should not satisfy ourselves with a statement like: This is "typical" for a patient recovering from an operation, the blood pressure is normal and, therefore, the condition of his circulation has to be stable.

It is our obligation to observe the action of catecholamines after injury and operation and to evaluate by improved diagnostic measures up to which point their action may be expedient and beneficial and to act immediately when we find the most essential criterion of shock: Persistence of ineffective peripheral circulation causing inadequate perfusion.

---

* Dr. AHNEFELD is ass. Professor of Anaesthesiology at the Institute of Anaesthesiology of the University of Mainz.

e) Sympathomimethic drugs and their relation
to the catecholamines

R. Kucher

The catecholamines and related substances have a direct effect on the
reacting cells. Substances with an effect similar to that of NE. are usually
designated as Symp.-drugs and, by release of NE., they act "indirectly".
As early as 1910, BARGER and DALE found that there is a number of "symp.
amines" which are very similar in their effect to E. The best symp. effect is
established by the arrangement of two phenolic hydroxyl groups in 3,4
position with regard to the side-chain (E., = Epinephrine, NE., = Norepinephrine, corbadrine, adrenon, isuprel). Substances without these hydroxyl-
groups are less effective and such substances with ephedrin-structure are differ-
entiated from those with a structure similar to epinephrin, by greater stability,
oral compatibility, a longer effect, as well as by their central component of effect
(ephedrin, norephidrin, amphetamine, methedrine, methoxamine). The effect
of a stimulation of the cerebrum is most marked in the case of amphetamin and
methedrine. Those substances containing only one phenolic hydroxyl-
group (synephrine, neosynephrine, pholedrine, etc.) have an intermediate
position between E. and ephedrin. The introduction of an alcoholic hydro-
xyl-group into the side-chain, usually increases the effect of the substance.
This is one of many possibilities of classifying symp. amines systematically.
In case of a restriction to symp. amines with purely vasopressoric effect, the
vasopressors are best classified according to those which release NE., those
which have similarity to E. and those which are neither similar to E. not to
NE. The first mentioned classification, however, seems more adequate to
me, with regard to anaesthesiology, as it best reflects their pharmacodynamic
efficiency, depending on the structure of the individual substances, so that
the indication of their use in anaesthesiology and resuscitation is determined.
Thus, please permit me to make some remarks being of interest with regard
to anaesthesiology, concerning the question of symp. drugs and their relation
to the catecholamines. I do not wish to discuss here in detail the special place
which is occupied by E. among the numerous symp. amines. It was and will
be dealt with sufficiently in other items of this discussion. With regard to
this specific question, the difference is biggest between ephedrin, which has
no effect, if the sympathetic ends of the nerve fibres are destroyed, and E.
which has an effect on the de-nerved organ also. But there are also manifest
differences in respect of the pharmacologic efficiency between corbadrine
and E., although they are chemically very similar.

Corbadrine has a strong vaso-constrictive effect and is one of the strongest
symp. amines, without increasing the medium blood pressure. It causes
significantly less side effects than E. We shall deal with this substance in the
section "Use and . . .".

Isuprel: has a 5–10 times stronger broncholytic effect than E. In contrast to most symp. amines it has a distinct vasodilatoric effect which reduces the peripheric resistance of the vessels. The usual depressor reply to isuprel may be transformed into a pressor-effect by administering symp. amines. This isuprelvasomotor-reverse effect cannot be achieved by NE. and is possibly antagonized. Isuprel develops a stimulating effect on the heart and, in contrast to E., it effects the sinus nodes and not the ventricular impulse centers. The experiment proves that Isuprel, in the case of a direct perfusion of the sinus nodes, triggers a sinus-tachycardia ten times smaller than that caused by E. and NE. Isuprel has a good effect in the case of bronchial asthma, postop. respiratory insufficiency, as a consequence of broncho-spastic disturbances, and in cases of mechanical artificial respiration of long duration, however, the tachycardia effect sets a limit to its use. An even more favorable effect may be achieved in the above described cases by *alupent* – only a change of the phenolic hydroxyl groups from the 3,4 to the 3,5 position – particularly in the case of transitory disturbances of the heart, such as total and partial Av-block. Moreover, there is more scope for the administration of long-term artificial respiration, on account of the smaller tachycardia effect. Of the symp. amines with a phenolic hydroxyl group, *synephrine* had a certain importance from the point of view of anaesthesiology, however, it was justly more and more superceded by NE. which, if the dosage is adequate, is superior to synephrine with regard to most components of its effect. It is only of a certain interest for the treatment of the somewhat indefinite concept of "general vascular atonia" and of vagally conditioned arrhythmia perpetua. The same applies to *neosynephrine* for the treatment of paroxysmal tachycardia which, however, in case of an over-dosage, causes ventricular extrasystoles and ventricular tachycardia, the same as E. does. *Pholedrine* has a similar effect as synephrine, the former having a longer effect. *Norpholedrine* and *metaradrine*, which peripherically have about the same effect as ephedrine, but have no centrally stimulating effect, should also be mentioned.

Of the symp. amines without a phenolic hydroxyl group, *Ephedrin* is of greatest interest. Its effect on the circulation is very similar to that of E., only a 100 times larger dosis is necessary. The effect, however, sets in slowly and lasts for 2–3 hours. As E., ephidrine stimulates the secondary centres of impulse formation in the ventricles. Even therapeutical doses may cause arrhythmias. The tachycardia effect is particularly strong. A direct perfusion of the sinus node causes a 10 times stronger sinus-tachycardia than the catecholamines and a ten times longer duration of the tachycardia. Moreover, the symp. drugs without a hydroxyl group in the benzene ring have, in contrast to the catecholamines, a distinct central stimulating effect which, especially in the case of fearful patients, leads to nervousness, fear, tremor, and anxiety. In this respect *norephidrin* is said to be more compatible. This far-reaching similarity of the pharmaco-dynamic effects of ephidrin and those of E. have made the use of ephidrin in anaesthesis recede into the background, as compared with NE. More about this in the section "Use and . . .".

Benzedrine (amphetamine) and *methedrine* have effects on the circulation which are, in general, similar to those caused by E. and stimulate the Central Nervous System even more than ephedrine does. This selective central stimulating effect, without an undesired circulatory effect, may be achieved by the use of a monoaminooxydasis block, which prevents the release of NE. out of the atria. For the anaesthetist, these substances have only a certain significance for the treatment of poisoning with sleeping drugs or testing the excitability of the cerebral cortex. *Methoxamine* shows almost no central stimulating effects, and is characterized by an almost exclusively pressoric effect. In contrast to NE., E., Synephrine, and other symp. amines, it only slightly impedes the efficiency of the cardiac muscle and does not influence the impulse-transmission system of the heart. On the other hand, an increase in blood pressure, as in the case of NE. may trigger a reflectively moderate bradycardia. In Europe, this substance is frequently used, in order to counteract a blood pressure decrease in spinal anaesthesia. The importance of symp. amines for intra-operative anaesthesia, as well as for after-treatment and resuscitation has clearly decreased during the last few years. The development ran almost parallel to the increasing interest in catecholamines, in particular as NE. has become better known. This is no chance development. In his heart of hearts the anaesthetist usually did not feel at ease when administering a symp. drug, and often, though not always, he considers it a sudden disturbance of the steady state. Because frequently, even today, anaesthetists administer a symp. drug to correct, mostly avoidable, anaesthesiologic, circulatory, or even respiratory disturbances, and then have to realize that the desired effect is not achieved. Why, even for the treatment of shocks symp. drugs are recommended and used, although there are no theoretical relations between the patho-physiology of the shock and the pharmaco-dynamic activity of the symp. drugs. Without running the danger of being called a "sympatholytic", I believe that catecholamines can only be granted a safe indication in the treatment of shocks, in specific pathogenetic forms, and here only in certain moments, in the course of the individual phases of the shock. However, Dr. FREY will give us detailed information about this. Please excuse my rather long talk, I will be briefer in the next section.

f) Catecholamines and shock

F. W. Ahnefeld and R. Frey

Catecholamines cause intense vasoconstriction which constitutes a fundamental body response at the beginning of shock. Their action is, therefore, in this way – and at this moment – lifesaving as an emergency reaction.

A disturbed relation of heart minute volume to peripheral demand indicates the beginning of decompensation which is characterized by metabolic disturbances.

Hereafter the effects of catecholamines can not be interpreted to be favorable any more since further vascular centralization will be followed by diminished peripheral perfusion and ensuing changes will influence the further course of shock and its therapy. This self-perpetuating course of shock is the reason why poor peripheral circulation may persist and volume substitution alone does not succeed if it is not started early enough, although it still remains the foundation of shock therapy. In these cases normalization of haemodynamics can only be achieved by simultaneous therapy with sympathicolytic drugs and volume substitution. Since we realize that shock is more a problem of perfusion and not of blood pressure alone! The amount of substitution ought to be estimated more by criteria for sufficient peripheral circulation than arterial blood pressure.

Our interpretation was confirmed in 2 series of studies.

In 20 burn cases we found a volume deficit from 12% to 34% within the first 3 hours, depending on the extent and severity of the injury.

It was most striking that

1. Blood pressure stayed within normal limits, sometimes even slightly elevated, in spite of hypovolemia and

2. Patients with a deficit of only 12% to 20% of the circulating volume – which in itself is not dangerous – showed typical signs of poor peripheral circulation already. At this time urine production, too, was below the critical amount of 25 ml/h.

From this 2 conclusions can be drawn in regard to therapy:

1. Aterial blood pressure alone is not a reliable criterion and its isolated consideration must lead to grave errors in diagnosis and also in the assessment of fluid substitution.

2. Impairment of capillary perfusion can occur with a relatively small decrease of circulating volume already.

An increased output of catecholamines is responsible for this discrepancy. Measurement of adrenalin and noradrenalin levels, when done within the first 3 hours concomitantly with volume determinations, showed an increase of 10 to 35 times of the norm in untreated burn patients. Complete normalization could not be achieved in the first 24 hours even with a sufficient supply of liquids. A reduction of the circulating volume of more than 10% – clinically hardly recognizable but affirmed by volume determination with the Volemetron (J^{131}-albumin) – led to a concurrent and significant increase of plasma catecholamine values.

Adrenalin and noradrenalin play an important role at the very beginning of shock in burn cases and other severe injuries. Their action, increased vasoconstriction, renders diagnoses and therapy difficult and is responsible for early derangement of metabolism. Poor capillary perfusion leads to acidosis with pH values at or below 7,2 in untreated burns after 1 to 2 hours already. Increasing amounts of lactic acid now stimulate the adrenal glands additionally.

It is this vicious circle which can not be interrupted by volume substitution alone. The excessive effect of catecholamines can cause damages within the first 24 hours which may manifest themselves after several days only.

g) Discussion

W. Fill

Die Rolle der Katecholamine bei der Anaesthesie und chirurgischem Eingriff ist bedeutend: Sie bewirken eine Mobilisierung der Abwehrkräfte über das sympathische System, die erwünscht und notwendig ist.

Andererseits wissen wir, daß Gefäßwände und Herzmuskel eine besondere Affinität zu Katecholaminen besitzen, und daß diese wahrscheinlich einen Einfluß auf die Entstehung arteriosklerotischer Veränderungen haben [Lit. bei Raab, Medizinische (1959), (p. 500–504) und Medizinische (1957), (p. 1–8). Pippig, Schneider, Hochrein, Mediz. Klin. (1962), (p. 1475 bis 1481)].

Sicher ist wohl, daß die Anwesenheit und der Abbau der Katecholamine den Sauerstoffverbrauch der Gewebe, also neben anderen den des Herzmuskels, steigern was im Stress eine Hypoxie desselben hervorrufen kann.

Diese schädlichen Nebenwirkungen der unvermeidlichen und sogar wünschenswerten sympathikotonischen Reaktion der Narkose und Operation kann vielleicht verhindert werden, wenn man die Fixierung der Katecholamine im Herzmuskel und den Coronargefäßen verringert.

Segontin (Synadrin), bekannt als Mittel zur Behandlung der Angina pectoris und des Herzinfarktes, verringert die Fixierung der Katecholamine im Herzen, den Gefäßen, den Halsganglien und im Gehirn, ohne jedoch die sympathikominetische Reaktion zu verhindern, wie das im stärkeren Maße die Rauwolfia-Präparate tun (Schöne und Lindner, Klin. Wschr. 1962, p. 1196.

Daher besteht die Möglichkeit, den schädigenden Einfluß der Katecholamine auf das Herz beim Stress der Anaesthesie und Operation zu verringern, was unter dieser speziellen Fragestellung untersucht werden sollte.

II. Praxis and application

a) Catécholamines dans l'hypothermie et l'hibernation provoquée

L. Lareng

Si le cortex surrénal a été depuis longtemps l'objet de travaux à l'origine de nombreuses applications à l'Anesthésie et à la Réanimation, les connaissances concernant la médullo-surrénale sont plus récentes étant données les difficultés à les expliquer biologiquement. Les dosages des catécholamines, récents, ont entr'autres permis une meilleurs application de la fonction médullo-surrénalienne en hypothermie.

Dans l'Hypothermie: L'activité de la médullo-surrénale des hibernants a été très étudiée; cependant les résultats n'ont pas toujours été concordants.

Pour ADLER, KAYSER et ARON une réduction de la sécrétion médullo-surrénale se produit pendant l'hibernation. Par contre, pour SUOMALINEN et UUSPAA se produit une augmentation du taux sanguin des catécholamines surrénaliennes au cours de l'hibernation, puis survient une brusque diminution de celles-ci au cours du réveil printannier (ceci ayant été étudié sur le hérisson).

PETROVIC et DAVIDOVIC de Belgrade ont réalisé en 1952, sur un lot important de spermophiles une série d'expérimentations en réalisant 5 lots de ces animaux pris à diverses périodes de l'hibernation.

Lot 1 – Animaux pris en début d'hibernation soit en novembre.

Lot 2 – Animaux ayant hiberné plusieurs mois et étudiés en janvier.

Lot 3 – Animaux ayant été maintenus artificiellement à une température élevée de 28 à 30° et sacrifiés en janvier sans avoir hiberné.

Lot 4 – Animaux ayant hiberné, et pris juste avant le réveil spontané en mars.

Lot 5 – Animaux ayant hiberné et pris après le réveil en avril.

Chez ces spermophiles, on étudie, d'une part le poids des surrénales exprimé en mg/100 gr de poids du corps et d'autre part, la teneur en catécholamines de celles-ci après extraction des catécholamines par le HCl à 0,02 N. Le taux des catécholamines est évalué par l'action plus ou moins importante de celles-ci sur la TA d'un rat traité par l'hexaméthonium et anesthésié à l'uréthane.

Le poids des surrénales des animaux en hibernation prolongée (lot 2) dépasse celui des animaux en début d'hibernation (lot 1). En mars on constate une faible diminution du poids des glandes (lot 4) et une forte augmentation autour du réveil printannier (lot 5).

Le taux des catécholamines par contre diminue au cours de l'hibernation prolongée par rapport à celui constaté en début d'hibernation (lot 1). Au printemps, juste avant le réveil, on note une forte accumulation de catécholamines dans la glande (lot 4) suivie d'une chute très nette après le réveil (lot 5).

Si l'on compare le taux des catécholamines des spermophiles du lot 2 et 3, ces derniers ont un taux supérieur; la fréquence des réveils spontanés des spermophiles a pour conséquence une diminution du taux des catécholamines; en effet le réveil provoque une hypersécrétion médullo-surrénalienne et la glande, pendant le sommeil qui suit n'est pas capable de rétablir l'état précédent. D'ailleurs c'est au moment du réveil que l'on trouve le taux le plus bas.

Pendant l'hibernation spontanée, nous constatons que le taux des catécholamines diminue progressivement dans la glande surrénale, mais leur sécrétion n'est jamais abolie.

Dans l'hypothermie provoquée: On a également étudié l'activité médullo-surrénalienne, après anesthésie (éther) et divers mélanges lytiques (réserpine) destinés à bloquer les réactions nocives dues au froid. Il semble que l'administration des drogues entraîne au début la stimulation des cellules phéochromes, et ce n'est que dans un deuxième temps, que l'on constate la baisse de leur activité.

Expérimentalement, chez le chien anesthésié à l'éther, on étudie:

a) – La réponse des glandes médullo-surrénaliennes provoqueés par un bain froid à 4°. Des modifications de l'activité médullo-surrénales, se produisent, se traduisant à la seule sécrétion paralytique observée après énervation de la glande lorsque la température centrale atteint 24–25°. L'effet ganglioplégique du froid s'exerce donc sur la synapse ganglionnaire qui représente la jonction médullo-surrénale. Ceci a été mis en évidence par Malmejac et son école, Hume et Egdhal, chez le chien. Brown et Cotten ont obtenus des résultats inverses alors que Fisher et Fedor n'ont pas constaté de modifications chez le rat.

b) – Ischémie médullo-surrénales et hypothermie: Si l'on continue d'abaisser la température centrale de l'animal (chien) au-dessous de 20° après arrêt circulatoire atteignant 45 à 60 minutes, il faut pour assurer la reprise de l'activité cardiaque deux lavages myocardiques. Le premier est destiné à rétablir les conditions physico-chimiques myocardiques favorables, le second à faire pénétrer l'adrénaline indispensable à la reprise du tonus cardiaque dans la circulation corronaire même. Il se produit alors une élévation tensionnelle telle, quelle ne peut être mise en totalité sur le compte du second lavage myocardique mais elle semble relever en partie comme c'est le cas en normothermie (après un bref clampage) de l'entraînement des catécholamines hypertensives d'origine médullo-surrénales accumulées durant l'hypothermie, avant l'arrêt complet de la sécrétion à 16°. Ceci a été mis en évidence par la technique dite de la « surrenale irriguée in situ » et corroboré par les dosages fluorimétriques.

On procède de la manière suivante: une surrénale est perfusée avec du sang rendu incoagulable, et dont la température varie de 38° à 16°. Bien qu'à la température de 18°, la glande se comporte comme énervée, MALMEJAC opère dans certains cas, sur des surrénales énervées. Le sang efférant est déversé chez un chien transfusé réactif, une partie de ce sang étant prélevée pour les dosages d'adrénaline et de nor-adrenaline suivant la méthode fluorimétrique.

On constate:

1 – Que le chien réactif, présente une hypertension importante, ainsi qu'une contraction des vaisseaux de sa rate, au moment du rétablissement de la circulation surrénale; des produits hypertenseurs d'origine surrénale ont donc été entraînés.

2 – Qu'il existe parallèlement un taux élevé d'amines hypertensives dont la proportion relative des deux catécholamines, adrénaline et nor-adrénaline, correspond à celle d'une sécrétion normale, à savoir 10% de nor -adrénaline, même si une sécrétion paralytique (20% de nor-adrénaline et plus) était bien établie au moment de l'ischémie.

On retiendra que si l'activité des cellules phéochromes diminue progressivement au cours de l'hypothermie provoquée pour être réduite à la sécrétion paralytique et être nulle à 16°, lors du réchauffement il y a reprise de l'activité surrénalienne ainsi que de l'ensemble du système adrénalinosécréteur. Cette reprise se manifeste dès 30° pour être à nouveau normale à 37°, même s'il y a eu ischémie pendant 45 à 60 minutes.

En conclusion en ce qui concerne le taux des catécholamines dans les surrénales on n'a pas retrouvé d'éléments absolument comparatifs entre l'animal hibernant, l'animal hiberné artificiellement, et l'homme. Ceci d'ailleurs ne saurait nous étonner car l'effet de l'hibernation se juge sur des mois.

Cependant, contrairement à l'hibernation spontanée, on constate que dans l'hibernation provoquée, on peut supprimer l'activité de la médullo-surrénale à condition de descendre à des températures très basses.

La sécrétion de la médullo-surrénale revient à un taux normal, lorsque la température de réchauffement atteint 37°. La relance cardiaque n'est possible que si l'on perfuse de l'adrénaline au cours du réchauffement entre 17 et 30°. De telles constatations permettent l'arrêt cardiaque prolongé sans danger pour la médullo-surrénale.

Bibliographie

Berther, A. and N. Millarps: Effect of reserpine on the storage of newformed catecholamines in the adrenal medulla. Acta Physio Scand. 1961, **52, 44.**

Bigelow, W. G. and S. Sidlofsky: Hypothermia and the effects of cold. British Medical Bulletin, 1961, **17,** 1.

Cenciotti, L. A.: Contribution to the study of artificial hibernation: 17 hydroxy and catecholamines in peripheral blood. Arcisped S. Anna Ferrara, 1959, **12,** 143.

Comisky, Mc: A note on metabolic effects of hypothermia in adrenalectomized rats. Canad. J. Biochimic Physiol. 1963, **41,** 2038.

Cooper: Physiology of hypothermia. British Journal Anesth. 1959, **13,** 96.

Hazard B. Beauvalet: Effets de la reserpine sur l'excrétion urinaire d'adrénaline et de nor-adrénaline chez le rat. Thérapie 1960, **15,** 692.

Holobut, W. and Coll.: The content of catecholamine hormon, adrenalin and nor-adrenaline in peripheral blood in moderate hypothermia. Acta Physiol. Polonof., 1963, **41,** 601.

Lofgren, L.: Reaction of adrenal contex during controled experimental hypothermia. Ann. med. exp. Fenn. 1963, **41,** 319.

Leblanc, J. A. et Nado, G.: Excretion urinaire d'adrénaline de et nor-adrénalin chez l'animal normal et l'animal adapté au froid. Canad. Journal Biochimic 1961, **39,** 215.

Lungarotti, F.: The sympathic ganglionic system in artificial hibernation. Minerva Chirurgica 1959, **14,** 1959.

Malmejac, J. Action de l'adrénaline sur le cœur du rat en hypothermie profonde. Lyon Médical 1963, **209,** 181.

Malmejac, J., Neverre, G., Bianchi, M. et Malmejac, Cl.: Ischémie médullosurrénalienne en hypothermie à 16–18°. Journal de Physiologie 1960, **52,** 162.

Malmejac, J., Malmejac, C., Laville, C., et Margarit, J. Action cardiaque de l'adrénaline en hypothermie profonde. C. R. De Société de Biologie 1963, **5,** 960.

Malmejac, J., Malmejac, C., Fredenussi, R., et Bonnet, D.: Resistance du système adrénalino-sécréteur à l'ischémie sous hypothermie contrôlée à 17–18°. C. R. Société de Biologie 1959, **2,** 1776.

Malmejac, J.: Action de l'adrénaline sur le cœur du rat en hypothermie profonde. Lyon Médical, 1963, **209,** 181.

Milar, R. A. and Morris, M. E.: Sympatho-adrenal reponse during general anaesthesia in the dog and man. Canada Anaesth. Soc. J. 1961, **8,** 356.

Perez Casa: Structural and histochimical variations in the adrenal gland of the dog rubmitted to the influence of artifical hibernation. Acta Histochimica 1961, **11,** 1–29.

Petrovic Davidovic: Effects of hibernation on the catecholamines levels of the spermophiles. C. B. Soc. Biolog. 1963, **7,** 1175.

Sellers, E. A.: Catecholamines in acclimatization to cold. Fed. Proc. 1963, **22,** 909.

Tohoku (Nagasaki): Effets de l'hypothermie sur le taux de la nor-adrénaline et de l'adrénaline de la médullo-surrenale du chat. Exp. Med. 1960, **71,** 70.

Warma, Gillis and Coll. On the relationship of catecholamines and tyroïde activity ot ventricular fibrillation during hypothermia in dogs. Canad. J. Biochim. 1963, **41,** 161

b) Use and abuse of catecholamines in local and regional anaesthesia

R. Kucher

It would go too far to speak in this context of the "use" of catecholamines in local anaesthesia. This would only be a systematic presentation of well-known facts which are dealt with in detail again and again periodically in textbooks, handbooks, and other publications. Thus, we would rather restrict ourselves to the "abuse" of catecholamines in local and regional anesthesia, but even so, it is only possible to deal with a few special questions.

Increase in the toxicity of the local anaesthetics by catecholamines and symp. amines: in the attempt to achieve a maximal bloodlessness in the area of the operation, or the longest possible effect in regional anaesthesia, many accidents are caused, because the quantity of catecholamines added is too big, thus leading to an indirect increase of the toxicity of the local anaesthetics. Such toxic symptoms account for 98% of all serious disturbances of local anaesthesia. As we may gather from recently published statistics by MOORE and BRIDENBAUGH, comprising 36000 cases of regional anaesthesias, toxic symptoms occur in 1.5% of the patients; in 0.3% of the patients there were serious signs of poisoning. Contrary to a still very common belief, the addition of vasoconstrictive substances does not reduce the toxicity of the local anaesthetics; there is no influence on the occurrence of complications. Catecholamines cause changes of metabolism and respiration, in accordance with the dose of these substances. The same applies to the changes of the circulation. KEIL deserves credit for the most exact investigation into the amount of increase in toxicity caused by E., and he was able to show that the toxicity of cocaine is increased by 240%, that of procain by 120–130%, that of pantocain by 100%, that of xylocain by about 100%, and that of nupercain by 400%. These recent experiments show how much smaller the lethal dosis is, if a catecholamine or carbadrine or another symp. drug is added to the salicain or oxyprocain.

Today we know a number of dangerous side effects of E. Its vasoconstrictive effect is only restricted to the vessels of the skin and the intestines. E. causes vaso-dilatation of the capillaries of the mucous membranes of the respiratory tract and the genital region, as well as of the urinary bladder.

This enables us to explain a number of unexplained accidents, some of them having been lethal which could not be cleared up so far and which occured after the use of a mixture of procain- or pantocain-E. for surface anaesthesia of the naso-pharyngeal area of the tracheo-bronchial system or of the urinary bladder. Therefore the addition of E. for surface anaesthesia in these areas is contra-indicated on account of the large resorption area caused by the dilatation of the capillaries. Neither is the resorption of the anaesthetic increased, nor is the duration of its effect longer. This statement also applies to other local anaesthetics, as well to NE. and other symp. amines. The reason for this is that the resorption of fluids from deeper airducts evidently takes place as quickly as in the case of an intravenous injection, the addition of E. having no influence on the resorption. E. causes a sensitization of the receptors, has a marked cardiac effect and finally acts in an intensifying way on the fissure products of the procain. One of these effector organ to E. and NE. As a rule, such accidents are not pure forms of fissure products, diethylaminoethanol, changes the susceptibility of the intoxication caused by the substance used for the local anaesthesia, or only a poisoning by catecholamines, but combination forms by a bilaterally induced increase of toxicity. Recent experiments have shown that cocaine retards the disappearence of circulating or free NE. and blocks the reception of NE. by the Schwann cells, thus increasing the effect of E. and NE. causing the addition of the exogenically introduced catecholamine which may result in undesired side effects or in an intoxication.

This possibility is particularly not sufficiently considered, if, for example, in the course of a general anaesthesia with cyclopropan or halothane, local anaesthetics with an addition of catecholamines are administered, not for the purpose of anaesthesia, but merely for the purpose of reducing bleeding and severing tissues in order to form „layers". This procedure is very frequently applied in oto-rhino-laryngologic operations, such as tonsillectomy, mucotomy, nasal septum operations, fenestration, etc., and in neuro – surgical and ophthalmologic operations. Many disturbances which occur in the case of cyclopropan- or halothan-anaesthesia in combination with local anaesthetics and the addition of catecholamines, that is, too large a dosis of catecholamines, might be prevented, if the pharmaco-dynamic interplay of these substances were known better.

Many contradictions may still be found in literature, however it may be considered a fact that already a cyclopropan anaesthesia as such leads to the release of catecholamines, that the operative trauma even increases this release, and that the heart reacts particularly easy to E. during the cyclopropan anaesthesia, with disturbances of the rhythm.

The pharmaco-dynamic conditions are somewhat different in the case of a halothane-anaesthesia, however, in the case of high concentrations it causes clinically similar disturbances. Sometimes they are even more serious, as the strong depressor effect of the halothane may lead to a stillstand of the heart rather quickly. The only reason why the frequency of the complications of this procedure has not become so drastically known in the world of medicine, is the enormous progress of the external cardiac resuscitation during the last years.

In these anaesthesia procedures, an exact, clinical, – I repeat clinical and not only electrocardiographic – cardiologic examination and a strict dosage of the catecholamine is indispensable. In this context, mention should be made of the erroneous and abusive use of catecholamines in spinal-and peridural-anaesthesia, for the purpose of preventing, respectively, above all treating a decrease in blood pressure. There is no objection to administering NE., which is preferable to ephedrin for various reasons, once, as a non-recurring addition to intra-muscular local anaesthesia in spinal-, respectively peridural anaesthesia. As we all know, we even should do it! But many patients would still be alive, if, in the case of a sudden hypotension in the course of a spinal- or peridural anaesthesia, instead of applying a catecholamine or a symp. drug, more attention would have had been paid to the blood volume, respectively the blood distribution. One may say that, apart from rare exceptions, after having administered NE. in the introductory local anaesthesia once, the administration of a catechol- or symp. amine in the course of a spinal or peridural anaesthesia, must be absolutely rejected. I do not even dare to discuss here the application of this method in the course of a general anaesthesia for the purpose of "correcting" variations in the blood pressure.

The intrathecal application of catechol, respectively symp. amines for the purpose of prolonging the effect of the spinal anaesthesia must also be judged with particular caution. We have a number of substances at our disposal today (nupercain, xylocain, etc.) which have a long-term effect; or the duration of the anaesthesia may be determined, if required by the continous spinal anaesthesia. I only wish to remind you of the increase of the toxicity of the local anaesthetics by catecholamines, – for example by 400% in the case of nupercain, apart from the specific effects of E. on the heart and the circulation.

Again and again we must point out the possibility of increasing and intensifying local damages (such as prolonged parasthesias, paralyses on account of necrosis in the region of the spinal cord and the cauda equina) by the addition of catecholamines.

Finally careless use of catecholamines in the course of infiltration-anaesthesia should be mentioned. Cutaneous necrosis, particularly in regions of disturbed circulation, as in arterio-sclerotic extremities, transplanted pedicled lobes, are attributed to the vaso-constrictive effect of NE., as the effect of NE., in this case, is more intense than that of E. In the case of an infiltration anaesthesia in the tissue with osseous basis (for example gum) apart from the vaso-constrictive component, the additional mechanically conditioned ischemia must also be taken into account. A number of things might still be mentioned, but I promised to be brief this time.

c) Use and compatibility of catecholamines during general anaesthesia

S. R. Oech

The use of catecholamines during general anaesthesia is rather limited. Of significance is the fact that their activity within the body may be influenced or modified by anaesthetics. Epinephrine and norepinephrine are extremely active biological substances, and it is likely that each compound is released to function in a specific body system.

Epinephrine. – Under normal physiologic conditions epinephrine is chiefly involved in locomotion and flight. It is primarily released into the circulation by the adrenal medulla in the form of an emergency hormone. An adequate stimulus for the release must be central in origin. This is obvious for apprehension, aggression, defense, and also pain which we have learned to regard as a function of the central nervous system. Some of the pharmacological effects are: positive chronotropic and inotropic action on the heart, vascular dilatation in sceletal muscle, bronchodilatation, and an increased state of alertness.

The liberation of epinephrine elicits an immediate maximal cardiovasuclar response. Such a response is non-specific and occurs during light anaesthesia with all anaesthetics as a reaction to noxious stimulation. Intubation in light anaesthesia, surgical incision in patients who are not adequately anaesthetized are stimuli which might fall into this category. With increasing depth, and in deeper planes of anaesthesia the activation of the emergency system becomes less, and is finally abolished.

Norepinephrine. – The introduction of the anti-hypertensive drugs, and also our better understanding of the mechanism of shock and hemorrhage have helped to clarify the role of norepinephrine. The amine serves as the humoral neurotransmittor of the adrenergic nervous system. It is present in every part of the circulatory system and released from adrenergic nerve endings, more analogous to acetylcholin than to a circulating hormone like epinephrine. Stores are ubiquitous. Cells with an ultra structure similar to that of chromaffin cells of the adrenal medulla were recently identified in the human dermis.

In man and animal the infusion of norepinephrine causes a rapid rise of the systolic, diastolic and mean arterial pressure with constriction of the peripheral vascular bed. To maintain the arterial pressure at a present hypertensive level requires constantly increasing amounts of drug. It may appear as if acute tolerance or refractoriness to the drug has developed. Peripheral resistance, however, remains high and the change is in the cardiac output. The cardiac output is markedly reduced, and one of the most important factors responsible for the reduction is a decrease of the circulating volume, mainly reduction of the plasma fraction. The absence of changes in the red cell mass eliminates the possibility of a portion of the circulating volume being trapped. The loss of plasma is explained by an increase in hydrostatic capillary pressure with changes of the pressure-filtration relationship across the capillary bed. FINNERTY and his associates and NICKERSON report reductions of 15 and 20 per cent respectively. If the infusion of norepinephrine is continued without the replacement of circulating volume shock will develop. At least one case of lethal iatrogenic shock produced by the prolonged administration of norepinephrine is documented in the literature.

If there is a causal relationship between increased amounts of norepinephrine and reduction in plasma volume, one would expect similar changes in patients with norepinephrine secreting tumors. Volumetric studies in patients with pheochromocytoma, indeed, have revealed reduced plasma volumes. Inversely, blocking of alpha receptors should result in an increase in circulating volume. The preoperative treatment with phentolamine reportedly did result in a return of the circulating volume to normal, and hypotension during operation and in the post-operative period did not occur.

The participation of norepinephrine in volume regulatory mechanisms also becomes evident during hemorrhage. FRANCIS D. MOORE bled normal volunteers. As soon as the circulating volume was reduced enormous amounts of catecholamines were found in the adrenal venous blood. Simultanously other compensatory mechanisms of the body to maintain homeostasis became operative. These included the secretion of aldosteron, renin, angiotensin, erythropoietin and conservation of sodium by the kidney. With the replenishment of he plasma volume by transcapillary refilling the outpouring of catecholamines ceased abruptly.

Under normal physiologic conditions norepinephrine is pharmacologically active in a homeostatic system which responds to changes in circulating volume, is capable of graded responses, and governed by a feed-back mechanism.

How is the situation during anaesthesia?

There are numerous reports which tend to show that the sympathetic nervous system performs a vital homeostatic function during anaesthesia by antagonizing the well known circulatory depressant effect of anaesthetics. The therapeutic use of drugs like reserpine which cause depletion of norepinephrine stores was believed to invite circulatory catastrophies during anaesthesia. After a single dose of reserpine maximal depletion occurs within 12–24 hours. Partial recovery takes place in 6–8 days, and restoration is complete after 10–20 days. A screening test to insure that adequate amounts of norepinephrine were present during operation, the ephedrine response test, was devised and abandoned as unreliable. In a clinical series KATZ, WEINTRAUB, and PAPPER compared untreated patients with those who had been on reserpine therapy from 6 months to 6 years prior to anaesthesia and surgery. These investigators found no difference in vascular responses during anaesthesia in the two groups. The consensus is that patient son reserpine therapy tolerate anaesthesia with all agents at least as well as patients whose body stores are not depleted of norepinephrine. Evidently, the mere fact that a person is undergoing anaesthesia does not cause an increased liberation of norepinephrine as an unspecific homestatic response.

Finally, specific effects of general anaesthetics have to be considered.

PRICE and his workers from the University of Pennsylvania found that with all anaesthetics studied the mean arterial pressure was best maintained during cyclopropane anaesthesia. Plasma concentrations of norepinephrine weresig nificantly elevated and also significantly related to anaesthetic concentrations. The cardiac output was elevated until end-expiratory concentrations of cyclopropane reached 17–21 per cent. With higher concentrations the cardiac output started to fall. In animals PRICE showed that these responses could be abolished after transection of the medulla oblongata at a level which removed the greater part of the medullary pressor center. By central nervous action then cyclopropane elicited a response similar to an infusion of norepinephrine. After extended administration of cyclopropane one would expect a reduction of the plasma volume with hemoconcentration. In addition, the reduction of the circulating volume might result in a precipitous fall in blood pressure once the administration of cyclopropane has ceased. Both effects are seen.

The same group of workers studied the circulatory effects of Halothane in normal man. The mean arterial blood pressure was reduced 28%, the vascular resistance was reduced 18%, and the average reduction of cardiac output and stroke volume was 15%. The oxygen consumption was reduced. Heart rate and venous pressure were unchanged. Catecholamine levels were essentially unchanged. The plasma volume was increased 11 per cent.

In animal experiments the mean arterial pressure, the contractile force of the heart, and the heart rate were found to be decreased when 1% halothane was admitted to the central nervous system only, but denied access to the rest of the body. The central action of the drug could be interpreted as suppression of sympathetic nervous activity, or possibly as a reduced responsiveness to cardiac and vascular smooth muscle to the sympathetic mediator, analogous to the effect of adrenergic receptor blockade. Accordingly, with this anaesthetic one would expect a transcapillary influx of water increasing the circulating volume. DEUTSCH, LINDE, DRIPPS, and PRICE found with progression in time and unchanged halothane concentrations a return of the cardiac output, blood pressure and heart rate to pre-anaesthetic levels.

Observation with other anaesthetics tend to show similar specific effects on the central nervous system in regard to sympatho-adrenal activation.

All anaesthetics which cause stimulation of the sympathetic nervous system predispose to cardiac arrhythmias. Present evidence favors the view that it is principally the liberation of excessive amounts of norepinephrine in the contracting syncytium itself which is responsible for the irregularities. There is a possibility that stimulation of cardiac sympathetic nerves can liberate norepinephrine in greater quantities than the myocardium is able to metabolize.

The fact that inhalation of carbon dioxide causes sympathetic nervous stimulation and arrhythmias is known and has been made use of in investigational work. By central action cyclopropane also causes the release of endogenous norepinephrine. In addition cyclopropane does not block the effects of carbon dioxide and these facts are held responsible for the occurrence of ventricular arrhythmias during cyclopropane anaesthesia.

PRICE and his co-workers have shown that an increase in alveolar CO_2-tension precipitated ventricular arrhythmias consisting of ventricular extrasystoles, bigeminal rhythm and multifocal ventricular tachycardia. In some of the subjects a very narrow threshold existed when the pCO_2 was increased without changing the endexpiratory concentration of cyclopropane. The threshold averaged 58 mmHg with a range of 44–72 mmHg. Catecholamine concentrations measured during the period of arrhythmia exeeded those before the period of hypercarbia. The return of the elevated pCO_2 to normal was usually associated with a return of the cardiac rhythm to normal together with a reduction of catecholamine levels. In several subjects the infusion of norepinephrine and epinephrine produced similar arrhythmias during cyclopropane anaesthesia. Measured concentrations in the plasma however were about ten times greater than during arrhythmias produced by hyperccarbia. Bilateral blockade of the stellate ganglion with local anaesthetics rendered hypercarbia practically ineffective in producing ventricular arrhythmias but did not significantly alter the ability of infused norepinephrine to do so. This suggests that endogenously released norepinephrine is responsible for the arrhythmias rather than circulating catecholamines.

KATZ, MATTEO und PAPPER studied the effects of injected epinephrine during general anesthesia. Half a miligram of epinephrine was injected in a solution of 1:60000 intramuscularly over a period of one hour. With halothane and trichloreoethylene the investigators found no significant difference between the injected group and the control group. With cyclopropane 11% of arrhythmias occurred in the control group. These were related to breath-holding, soft tissue obstruction, coughing etc. In the injected series they found 41% of arrhythmias, of which 30% were directly related to the injection of epinephrine. At the time when the arrhythmias occurred the pCO_2 was 44 mmHg or less.

Summary: The amount of endogenously released norepinephrine in the heart seems of greater significance in regard to the occurrance of arrhythmias than the level of circulating catecholamines. In animal, as well as in man the injection of a beta adrenergic receptor blocking agent, as dichloroisoproterenol, can prevent or abolish ventricular arrhythmias.

Chairman: I want to mention at this point the excellent paper read today by Michael Johnstone (Manchester). He was able to abolish anaesthesia induced ventricular fibrillation by β-receptor blockers (Anaesthesist **13**, 215, 1964).

d) Catecholamines in cardiac resuscitation

J. Beard

As a basis for discussion I want to mention some of the factors which seem important with regard to catecholamine effects on the heart and on it's resuscitation. Those familiar with work in this field will recognise the views of SARNOFF, BRAUNWALD and BURN, amongst many others.

The long refractory period of cardiac muscle, which distinguishes it from ordinary skeletal muscle, tends to discourage irregular contractions amongst the fibres which might otherwise lead to fibrillation. A long refractory period however apparently needs energy for its maintenance: in the absence of an adequate energy supply it seems that the duration of action potential is reduced and fibrillation made more likely. It is considered that one of the β stimulant effects of catecholamines is to increase the availability of energy to the heart muscle.

We must distinguish between atrial and ventricular muscle, since the ventricle has no parasympathetic innervation. In the isolated heart preparation, acetylecholine may lead to auricular fibrillation, and it is found that in this situation, adrenalin has a protective effect. It is presumed that this is due to extra energy made vailable for prolongation of action potential. Although it somewhat reduces cardiac output, atrial fibrillation is seldom of great concern to us in cardiac resucitation, and we will not consider it further.

In the ventricle, however, the situation is different since in the isolated heart, adrenalin not uncommonly leads to ventricular fibrillation. The explanation probably lies in the limited energy supplies available to the myocardium in the isolated perfused heart. In these circumstances there may well be insufficient energy both to increase the rate and force of contraction and to simultaneously maintain a long action potential-fibrillation therefore following administration. In the whole animal, energy is more likely to be available unless its liberation is prevented by noxious substances such as chloroform, and the force of contraction can be increased without simultaneous shortening of the action potential.

In the heart, nor-adrenalin exists in granules and vesicles which seem to be distributed in relation to sympathetic nerve fibres. The adrenalin is bound to A.T.P., four molecules of which combine with one molecule of adrenalin. From these vesicles, which can be demonstrated by electron microscopy and fluorescent staining, nor-adrenalin is released and taken up into the cell bodies where it exerts its characteristic action on sympathetic nerve stimulation. The immediate regulation of catecholamine activity in the heart seems to be dependant on sympathetic nervous system activity which regulates the release and uptake of nor-adrenalin from stores into the cells. The system is complex and seems to function in compartments. The enzymes concerned in catecholamine metabolism appear to have a long term, rather than immediate, effect on catecholamine levels, probably playing their major role in the viscera other than the heart.

Increased sympathetic activity increases the amount of nor-adrenalin released into the arterial blood. The average normal of 0.28 micrograms per litre rising to 0.46 or even 0.62 after really stenuous exercise. Heart disease without evidence of failure is not accommpanied by increased blood levels, but when heart failure occurs the level is comparable with that seen after stenuous exercise, exercise in the presence of heart failure leading to the highest figures seen 1.73. Those patients who have had heart failure are therefore subject to a depletion of myocardial catecholamines which can well be as great as occurs in those who have been treated with reserpine. (CHIDSEY, BRAUNWALD, et al., New England Medical Journal 1963, Vol. 269, Page 653.) Not that reserpine depletion is complete since some catecholamines can still be liberated by sympathetic nerve action even after prolonged administration of reserpine.

Catecholamine effects differ, the α receptor stimulators raising the peripheral resistance without direct effect on the heart, whereas the β receptor stimulators have a direct action on the heart muscle aiding glycogen breakdown. Not many substances act exclusively on one or other system, but the predominant action might well be kept in mind when selecting our drugs in cardiac resucitation. In the clinical conditions when cardiac arrest is likely to occur, oxygen and blood-born energy supplies are likely to be in short supply. Under these circumstances agents which increase the force and rate of the heart might well be expected to precipitate ventricular fibrillation. Later, when efficient cardiac compression and ventilation of the lungs have restored myocardial nutrition and oxygen supply, adrenalin, by releasing energy, may well help the action of the heart and assist in resuscitation. Furthermore agents which constrict the peripheral blood vessels will help by raising the blood pressure in the aorta, favouring a blood supply to the brain and coronary arteries. It must be remembered however, that this would be at the expense of many tissues, in which anaerobic metabolism must be expected to continue with the production of metabolic acidosis. This is an important factor since when it is present catecholamine action is notably depressed. Correction of metabolic acidosis by buffers or alkalis must therefore be regarded as an important part of cardiac resuscitation. In practice α stimulators have been found as effective as β stimulators in restoring cardiac action (PEARSON and REDDING 1963), which would seem to indicate that the maintenance of an efficient coronary filling pressure to provide cardiac nutrition is a factor of major importance.

Chairman: I want to thank you all very much indeed, the members of the panel for their excellent contributions and the audience for the interest and patience and the many questions asked.

Unfortunately, our time is limited and does not allow any discussion of further problems.

May I close with the following statement: It is our obligation to observe carefully the action of catecholamines after injury, operation and anaesthesia and to evaluate by improved diagnostic measures up to which point their action may be expedient and beneficial, and to act immediately (by infusion or transfusion and, if necessary, by adrenolytic drugs like Hydergin and some Phenothiazines), when we find the most essential criterion of shock: Persistence of ineffective peripheral circulation causing inadaequate perfusion.

III. References

(to: A. Catecholamines and their significance in anaesthesia)

AXELROD, J.: Enzymatic Formation of Adrenaline and other Catechols from Monophenols. Science **140**, 499 (1963).

BERTLER, A., CARLSSON, A., and E. ROSENGREN, E.: A Method for the Fluorimetric Determination of Adrenaline and Noradrenaline in Tissues I, Acta physiol. scand. **44**, 273–292 (1958).

BOOKER (1) and M. WALTER: The isolated Perfused Guinea Pig Heart as a Biological Assay Method for Adrenaline and Nor-Adrenaline (1) Arch. Internationales de Pharmacodynamie et de Thérapie Vol. CXXIII, Fascicule I–II, 206 (1959).

BRÜCKE, F., H. KNAUPP, B. OBENAUS, B. PILLAT und H. STORMANN: Der Einfluß möglicher Adrenalinvorstufen auf die Ausscheidung von Adrenalin im Harn von Ratten. Biochem. Pharmacology, **1**, 83–92 (1958).

BURN, J. H.: "The Cause of Fibrillation". Canadian Medical Association Journal. **840**, 625 (1961).

BURN, J. H. and M. J. RAND: The relation of circulating Noradrenaline to the effect of sympathetic stimulation. J. Physiol. (London) **150**, 295 (1960).

CARLSSON, A. and B. WALDECK: A Fluorimetric Method for the Determination of Dopamine (3-Hydroxatyramine). Acta physiol. scand. **44**, 293–298 (1958).

CHAPPEL, C.: Comparison of cardiotoxic actions of sympathomimetic amines. Canad. J. Biochem. **37**, 35 (1959).

CHIDSEY, C. A., BRAUNWALD, E., MORROW, A. G., and D. T. MASON: "Myocardial norepinephrine concentration in man". The New England Journal of Medicine. **269**, 653 (1963).

CRAWFORD, T. B. B. und W. LAW: Ausscheidung von Adrenalin und Noradrenalin im Rattenharn unter verschiedenen exp. Bedingungen. Brit. Journ. Pharmacol. **13**, 35 (1958).

CRAWFORD, T. B. B. and W. LAW: Method for the estimation of Adrenaline and Noradrenaline in urine, J. Pharm. (London) **10**, 179 (1958).

DE BLASI, SEBASTIANO: Association of alpha- and beta-receptor adrenergic blocking drugs in the anaesthetic management of patients with Phaeochromocytoma. Proc. III. World Congress of Anaesthesiology, São Paulo 1964, 128.

DE GENNES, MILLIEZ, BRICAIRE, QUICHAUD, LAUDAT, and MOUKHTAR, BAILLET: Les «Catécholamines Urinaires». Application du Dosage des catéchols-urinaires libres. Au Dépistage du Médulla-Suprénalome. Extrait de la Presse Médicale, 66. Année, **36**, 805–808 (1958).

DE SCHAEPDRYVER, A. F.: Differential Fluorimetric Estimation of Adrenaline and Noradrenaline in Urine. Arch. Internationales de Pharmacodynamie et de Thérapie, Vol. CXV, Fasc. I–II, 233 (1958).

DE SCHAEPDRYVER, A. F.: Differential Fluorimetric Estimation of Adrenaline and Noradrenaline in Plasma. Arch. Internationales de Pharmacodynamie et de Thérapie, Vol. CXVII, Fasc. III–IV, 475 (1958).

DILLER, W. F.: Faktoren, welche die biologische Bestimmung von Adrenalin im Urin stören und ihre Eliminierung. Ref. in Ron. Ber. **201**, 14 (1958) nach Arch. internat. Pharmacodynamie **114**, 92 (1958).

DUNDEE, J. W.: Alterations in response to somatic pain associated with anaesthesia. IX. The effects of Hypercarbia and Catechol Amines. British Journ. of Anaesthesia **34**, 24 (1962).

EULER, v., U. S. and F. LISHAJKO: The Estimation of Catechol Amines in urine. Acta physiol. scand. **45**, 122–132 (1959).

EULER, v., U. S. und J. ORWIN: Gewinnung von Adrenalin und Nor-Adrenalin im Urin. Acta Physiologicy Scand. **33**, 118 (1955).

FELLMANN, J. H.: A New Colorimetric Method for the quantitative Determination of Epinephrine and Norepinephrine. Arch. Biochem. Biophys. **85**, 345 (1959).

GADDUM und LEMBECK: Methode: I. v. Injektion von radioaktiv markiertem Adrenalin 1–5 % werden in biologisch wirksamer Form ausgeschieden (Hinweis).

GRABOW, L.: Mode of Action of Catecholamines with Regard to pH. Proc. III. World Congress of Anaesthesiology, São Paulo 1964, 137.

GRAY, C.: Haemorrhagic Shock and the Nervous System Amer. J. Surg. **106**, 233 (1963).

HELMER, O. M.: Estimation of Urinary Catechol amines by means of a strip of rabbit Aorta as an aid in the diagnosis of Pheochromocytoma. The Journal of Laboratory and Clinical Medicine, St. Louis, **50**, 5, 737–744 (1957).

HILTON, WEAVER, MUELHEIMS, GLAVIANO, and WÉGRIA: Perfusion of the Isolated Adrenals in Situ. The American Journ. of Physiology **192**, 3, 525 (1958).

HOFMAN-ZITO, S.: Casasbuenas-Ayala, J., Mudoz-Wustsher, G.: Nuevos Aspectos de los Simpaticomimeticos en Anestesia. Proc. III. World Congress of Anaesthesiology, São Paulo 1964, 149.

JONES, W. P. G., M. B., Ch. B., F.A.C.A.: Inborn Errors of Catecholamine Metabolism. Proc. III. World Congress of Anaesthesiology, São Paulo 1964, 140.

KÄGI: Modifikation zur Fluoreszenzmethode von Weil-Malherbe und Bom im menschlichen Blutplasma, Al_2O_3 Verarbeitung. Arch. exp. Path. u. Pharmak. **230**, 421 (1957).

KEENAN, P., P. KLEITSCH, and L. HUMOLLER: The Determination of Catechol Amines in Blood. Clinical Chemistry, **5**, 3, 239 (1959).

KNAUFF, H. G. und G. VERBEEK: Flurometrische Bestimmungen von Adrenalin und Noradrenalin im Harn. Ergebnisse bei Gesunden u. bei Patienten mit Hypertonus. Klin. Wschr. **40**, 18–23 (1962).

MILLAN, MARY: Urinary Excretion of Individual Catechol Detivatives. The Lancet XIV of Vol. I, 6971, Vol. CCLXXII, 715 (1957).

MILLAR, R. A. and T. J. BISCOE: Effect of Anaesthetics on Preganglionic Sympathetic Discharge. Proceedings III. World Congress of Anaesthesiology, São Paulo 1964, 120.

NICOLOFF, D. M., E. T. PETER, A. S. LEONARD and O. H. WANGENSTEEN: Catecholamines in Ulcer Provocation I.A.M.A. **191**, 383 (1965).

PEARSON, J. W. and J. S. REDDING: "The Role of Epinephrine in Cardiac Resuscitation". Anesthesia and Analgesia Current Researches. **42**, 569 (1963).

RAAB, W. u. W. GIGEE: Die Katecholamine des Herzens. Arch. exper. Path. u. Pharmakol. **219**, 248–262 (1953).

RESNICK, O. und F. ELMADJIAN: Bestimmung von Adrenalin und Noradrenalin im Harn. Ref. in Ron. Ber. 200, 243 (1958) nach J. Clin. Endocrin. a. Metabolism **18**, 28 (1958).

RITZEL, G. und W. A. HUNZINGER: Über die Bestimmung von Katecholaminen im Urin. Klin. Wschr. **41**, 9, 419–423 (1963).

ROBINSON, R.: Secretion of Catecholamines in Malignant Phaechromocytoma. Brit. Med. Journal 1964, 1, 1422–1424.

SCHAPIRO, SHAWN (1): Effect of a Catechol amine Blocking Agent (Dibenzyline) on Organ Content and Urine. Excretion of Noradrenaline and Adrenaline, Acta physiol. scand. **42**, 371–375 (1958).

SCHMIDT, E. und R. TAUGNER: Die Kreislaufwirkung von 29 sympathomimetischen Aminen am wachen Hund. Arzneimittel-Forschung **10**, 19 (1960).

SKALIKS, H. CH:. Der Nachweis einiger Sympathicomimetica auf Papierchromatogrammen. Arzneimittel-Forschung **7**, 386–387 (1957).

STEWART, NEWHALL, and EDWARDS: Ref. in Dtsch. Apothekerzeitung **104**, 995 (1964), nach J. biol. Chemie **239**, 930 (1964).

TYRER, J. H.: Die Wirkung von l-Adrenalin und dl-Noradrenalin auf den mittleren Druck der rechten Vorkammer des Schafes. Quart. J. exp. Phys. cognate med. Sci. **38**, 169 (1953).

VOGT, MARTHE: Drugs and Metabolism of Catecholamines in the Brain. British Medical Bulletin **21**, 57 (1965).

B. Clinical use of halogenated agents

Chairman: L. E. MORRIS, Seattle.
Members: J. F. ARTUSIO, New York; M. H. HOLMDAHL, Uppsala; M. W. JOHNSTONE, Manchester; W. W. MUSHIN, Cardiff.

Morris: First I would like to introduce my Panel, experts in their field, and who are all colleagues of yours on the international scene. To your right and my left, at the far end, is Dr. ARTUSIO, from the Cornell Medical Center, New York City. Dr. ARTUSIO has special interest in halogenated anaesthetic agents and particularly so in methoxyflurane. Next to him is Dr. MICHAEL JOHNSTONE, from Manchester, England, who is, as MAX SADOVE called him a year ago, the father of the clinical use of halothane. Next to him and next to me is Dr. MARTIN HOLMDAHL, from Sweden. We are very pleased to have him here to act as the devil's advocate; to challenge the ideas which are expressed upon this Panel by some of the others. To my right and your left is Dr. WILLIAM MUSHIN, from Cardiff, also an authority in the halogenated anaesthetics. We are particularly delighted to have him on this Panel because he is among those who have recently been moved to conduct detailed retrospective studies of the effects of halothane upon various systems of the body.

Now, there should be among you, distributed up and down the tiers here, some bits of paper upon which to write questions for submission to the Panel. We want to use your questions; we want you to know that this is to be a spontaneous discussion, an unrehearsed Panel, which in effect will not succeed unless you ask us questions. So, would you please then prepare your questions and have one of the young ladies bring them down to us, so that we may do our best to give you some discussion of questions.

Now, during the past ten years, the pharmacologists and pharmaceutical houses have actually introduced to our use a number of fluorinated compounds which purport to have some special benefits. We hope to elucidate some of these and to draw from the Panel Members what they think about some of these agents. Three of these agents – halothane, fluoromar and penthrane – have achieved some popularity in the intervening years, and I think it would be well for us to ask the basis for that popularity. Certainly we should not follow the lead of the enthusiasts unless we have good foundation and good reasons for using these agents in place of something else.

We will then begin by asking the Panel Members each to tell us his idea as to why the halogenated anaesthetic agents are useful and have, in a part at least, usurped a rightful place from other techniques and agents with which we had come to have some familiarity. I will begin with Dr. Mushin, on your left.

Mushin: Mr. Chairman, the two halogenated anaesthetics to which my remarks will apply are trichlorethylene and fluothane. These are the two which have been introduced during the period which we call modern anaesthesia. I think there are three basic reasons why they have become so popular. First and foremost, because they are non-flammable. Secondly, because they are powerful. And thirdly because, in producing their anaesthetic effects, they are in general also cardiovascular depressants. Blood pressure tends to fall and the operation area becomes attractively ischaemic. Now, these are the three characteristics which I think explain their popularity. Fluothane quite certainly was deliberately sought for and deliberately introduced into anaesthesia to supply a non-flammable anaesthetic alternative to ether.

Morris: I think we have returned to inhalation agents because of their relative safety and the ease of adjusting the anaesthetic effects from moment to moment, according to need and according to the biological variation in response. Dr. Holmdahl, would you like to add?

Holmdahl: I would just like to say that we need, under some circumstances, a powerful inhalation anaesthetic agent. Some centers may say that we just need nitrous oxide-oxygen and a relaxant agent. We just have to try to give anaesthetics high up in Bogota, Columbia, to understand that you cannot always anaesthetize a patient that way. Therefore we need safe, flexible, and potent inhalation anaesthetic agents so that you can have a distinct level of anaesthesia without interfering too much with the available oxygen. I would like to come back to that later. In addition, a good agent provides less secretion, good possibility for control of ventilation, and little depression of cardiac output; that is what we look for when we look out for a new potent inhalation anaesthetic agent . . .

Morris: Dr. Johnstone, would you like to add to these comments?

Johnstone: Yes. Well, my interest in halothane began about eight years ago and was provoked primarily because I thought the existing methods of anaesthesia at that time were too dependant on polypharmacy; many drugs of different pharmacological actions given intravenously for different indications; narcosis maintained mainly by nitrous oxide and often with complete paralysis of patients. I found that this method, although it had its uses and was quite effective, was rather complicated and virtually impossible to teach in an objective manner to undergraduate students. I thought, at the time, that this was perhaps bringing undergraduate teaching to a standstill – as it actually had in some places. (To me that seems a rather suicidal policy as regards the future of anaesthesia.) I felt, as my knowledge of halothane increased, that halothane might perhaps restore a logical attitude toward undergraduate teaching and thereby increase the numbers of medical practitioners who will take up anaesthesia after qualification. Other interests of course came along as time went on – pharmacological, academic, clinical, and so on – in relation to this particular drug which has maintained my interest up to the present time.

Morris: Dr. ARTUSIO, would you like to add something here? And since the others have been talking mostly about fluothane, perhaps you would mention some of the other agents?

Artusio: Well, certainly. Our interest in the halogenated anaesthetics began when we were seeking safety in new anaesthetic agents. We attempted to find a so-called super nitrous oxide type of gas, where the biologic potency of the compound would be greater than nitrous oxide, and whose absolute potency was in the range of approximately fifty volumes percent. It was our contention that much of the cardiac arrest associated with the induction phase of anaesthesia was iatrogenic. In the achievement of adequate alveolar ventilation, extremely potent agents are literally pushed into patients until they sustain acute myocardial overdose. Our intention, therefore, was to develop a drug in which maximum ventilation would be accomplished without the danger of anaesthetic overdose. At that time, one of the physiologists at Cornell was working with peripheral nerves, testing the genetrons and freons (commercial refrigerants) on these structures. He indicated to us that these agents might be useful in our field of investigation. This is the reason why we began to study the halogenated compounds. Although we did not find the super nitrous oxide gas we sought, we found a compound of the ether series which had, built within the molecule, the safety factor for which we were looking. This safety factor was related to the low saturated vapour pressure of the compound.

The drug methoxyflurane was picked for extensive clinical trial, based a good deal upon this safety factor. This is how our interest developed in the field of fluorinated hydrocarbons and ethers, and the reason why we chose methoxyflurane.

Morris: Well, that is a good beginning. Now, in view of Dr. ARTUSIO comments, I think it might be well to immediately ask the Members of the Panel how the physical properties of inhalation anaesthetics actually determine anaesthetic effects. Would you like to start that part of the story, Dr. MUSHIN?

Mushin: Table 1 pinpoints the main issue and, if the meaning of this simple table is understood, recent advances in this field become clear. Here are contrasted three common anaesthetics: ether, which has a high blood solubility and a fairly low fat solubility; halothane, which has a low blood solubility but a high fat solubility; and methoxyflurane, which has a blood solubility of the same order as ether, but a very high fat solubility. The solubility in water or in blood determines how quickly the arterial blood comes into equilibrium with the inhaled concentration. With ether, which has a high blood solubility, induction is slow because the blood carries away the ether vapour from the alveoli so fast that its partial pressure remains rather low. Hence induction is slow in the case of an anaesthetic vapour which is very blood soluble. On the other hand, in the case of a vapour which is not very soluble, induction is fast. Induction of anaesthesia using methoxyflurane is very slow because of its high blood solubility.

Table 1. *Blood/gas and fat/gas partition coefficients at 37° C*

	Solubility in Blood	Induction	Recovery from Short Op.	Solubility in Fat	Recovery from Very long Op.
Ether	15 +	slow	slow	50 −	slow
Halo-thane	2.3 −	fast	fast	138 +	slow
Methoxy flurane	13 +	slow	slow	825* + +	very slow

* Editor's Note: This is solubility in oil; solubility in fat is 0.60 × oil solubility = 495. (Ref. – EGER, E. I., and SHARGEL, R. – The solubility of methoxyflurane in human blood and tissue homogenates. Anaesthesiology **24**, 625–627 1963).

During recovery from the anaesthesia, we see the same thing in reverse, an exact mirror image of the same process. It is only when surgery has been going on for a very long time, that the effect of fat solubility comes into operation. In the case of halothane, recovery is then slower, but with ether, which is not very fat soluble, there is hardly any additional effect on the recovery time, which is almost the same as the induction time. In the case of methoxyflurane, however, if the operation goes on for a long time, recovery will be very slow indeed.

Fig. 1 has been drawn as the result of computations by the use of an electronic analogue computer developed by my colleague, W. W. MAPLESON, PH. D., in my Department. This computer is an electrical model of the body systems, and imitates the transport of the anaesthetic vapour from the alveoli into the blood stream, and from there to the various organs of the body, and so on back to the expired air. On the vertical axis of the graph is the recovery time on the logarithmic scale, and on the horizontal axis is the duration of administration also in the form of a logarithmic scale. On the right are concentrations of anaesthetic remaining in the brain, as percentages of what was there during anaesthesia. In other words, "10%" means nearly full recovery (90% recovery). Now, we did not know how to interpret those percentage figures until an article appeared by LINDSLEY, et al., in which he made some observations. These are shown as crosses and circles. To cut matters short, the "30%" line indicates what clinical anaesthetists would call "initial" recovery, i.e., to the point at which the patient responds to stimuli. With reference to the 30% line, so long as the duration of anaesthesia is up to one hour, the recovery line from halothane is almost horizontal. In other words, it does not make much difference whether the operation lasted ten minutes or one hour, or even two hours.

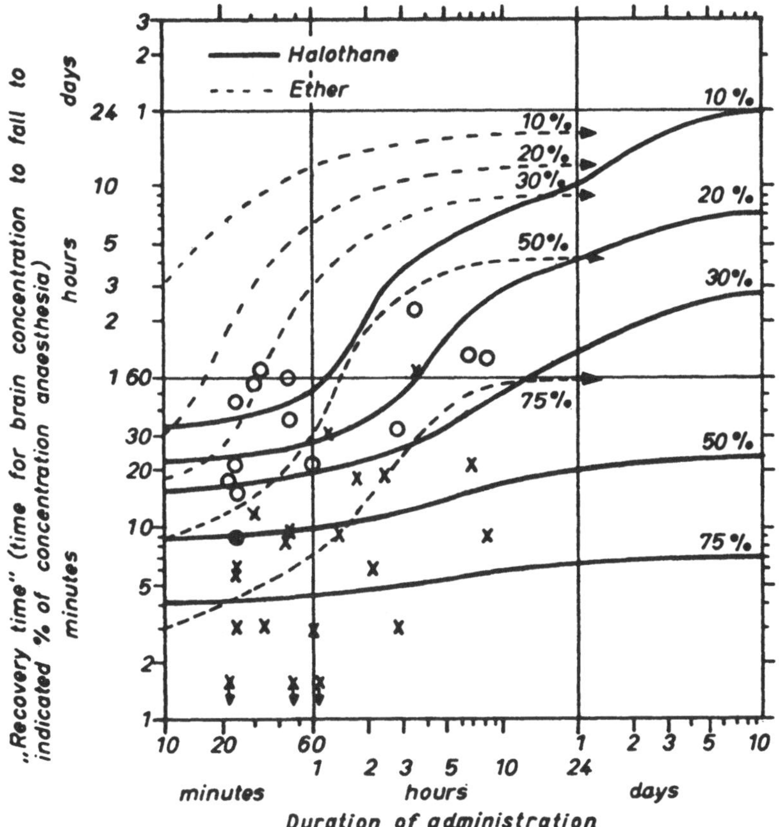

Fig. 1. (Fig. 6–7). Recovery Time versus Duration of Administration, x = 'Initial', O = 'Full', recovery from halothane in patients (LINDSLEY et al.: Anesthesiol. 22 [1961] 937). Copied from "Uptake and Distribution of Anesthetic Agents", Papper and Kitz, 1963. (Chapter by W. W. Mapleson).

The dotted curves are for ether, and these are very different because, in that period of up to two hours, the ether "30%" line is rising very steeply. Recovery after a ten-minute operation is somewhere about ten minutes, but at the end of one hour the recovery period is about one hour. This fits in with clinical experience that, within ordinary lengths of surgery of up to about one hour or one-and-a-half hours, recovery from fluothane is fairly rapid, whereas the duration of anaesthesia makes a very big difference in the case of ether.

Morris: Thank you very much. Now we have started talking about physical factors that have to do with how anaesthetics work and, I think, before we proceed much further, we should get Dr. MUSHIN and Dr. JOHN-STONE to engage in a little discussion of the factors which may be concerned with control of concentration of anaesthetics that we use. Now, I feel very strongly that moment-to-moment changes in concentration offered to the patient are most important while these two gentlemen tend to feel that we should be more interested in the total amount, total volume of agent which is put out per unit time and actually taken in by the patient. Now, I am sure that the truth encompasses some of both these points of view. I think, how-ever, that we need to hear from Dr. JOHNSTONE now, as to why he thinks that it may be just as safe to use a closed system as it is to use a high flow where one has better control over the actual percentage concentration.

Johnstone: I think the closed system of anaesthesia is probably the safest, the most controllable and the most economic, provided the vaporizer is outside of the circuit, and one constantly measures the amount of fluo-thane vapour in cubic centimeters per minute which one is feeding into that circuit, and therefore exposing one's patient to. The vaporizer inside the circuit of course is quite a different kettle of fish; it is being used success-fully, but the user has absolutely no idea as to the amount of halothane which he is giving at a particular moment. On the open systems with high flows, non-rebreathing methods, semi-open and so on, the anaesthetist again has no idea how much halothane is given, even from a calibrated vaporizer, unless he also is actually measuring the minute volume of the patient. Therefore, I would say that concentration is only half the story, half the information which one actually needs. It would be as silly to say that I gave 1% fluothane as it would be to say that I gave 1% pentothal to the patient. It gives one no idea of dosage received by the patient.

Morris: Dr. MUSHIN, would you like to carry on along this line of thought?

Mushin: I am really in full agreement with my colleague, Dr. JOHN-STONE, but we express our ideas in a rather different way. I prefer to keep to a mode of expression with which anaesthetists are perhaps more familiar.

I do not really think it matters by what method you make up the mixture wich the patient inspires, so long as you have some idea of both the concentration of the mixture and the ventilation of the patient. This gives you the same information as Dr. JOHNSTONE was indicating.

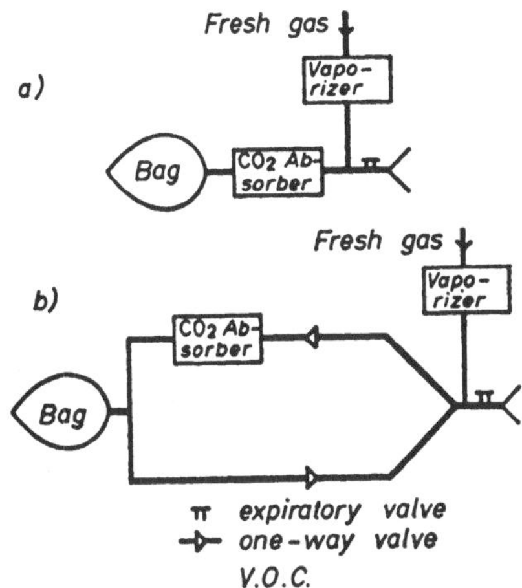

Fig. 2. (V.O.C.) Vaporizer Outside the Circuit. Mapleson, W. W. – Brit. J. Anaesth., 1960, **32**: 298.

I am not sure that everybody here is quite clear as to what we mean by the two terms, "V.I.C." and "V.O.C." In Fig. 2, the diagrams show quite clearly that the vaporizer is outside the breathing circuit, the breathing circuit being in one case a to-and-fro absorber system and in the other a circle system. This is called the V.O.C. – the Vaporizer Outside the Circuit. In Fig. 3, the Vaporizer is Inside the Circuit. This is called the V.I.C.

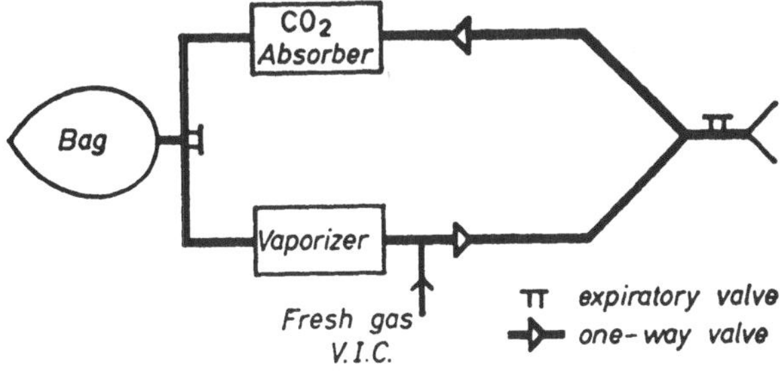

Fig. 3.(V.I.C.) Vaporizer Inside the Circuit. Mapleson, W. W. – Brit. J. Anaesth., 1960, **32**: 298.

Fig. 4 indicates the relationship between what is indicated on the vaporizer and what the patient inhales. If there is a completely non-rebreathing circuit, with a valve or other means which prevents rebreathing, then the

diagonal indicates that the indicated concentration on the vaporizer will
be exactly what the patient inhales. The left hand line is what happens if
an absorption system is used with the vaporizer inside the circuit. In this

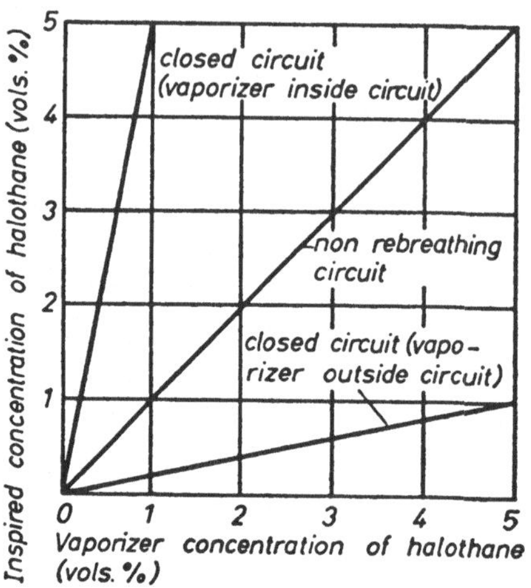

Fig. 4. Relationship between concentration on vaporizer and concentration inspired by
patient (for closed circuits: Ventilation = 5 l/min fresh gas flow = 0.2 l/min Oxygen).
Mapleson, W. W. – Brit. J. Anaesth., 1960, 32: 298.

situation (V.I.C.), whatever is indicated on the vaporizer, the patient will
always inhale a stronger concentration. How much stronger depends on
both the ventilation of the patient – a very important factor – and also on
the volume of fresh gas flow. The lower line at the bottom shows what
happens when the vaporizer is outside the circuit. Here, whatever is indicated on the vaporizer, the patient will always inhale something less than
that indicated on the vaporizer. The amount less, again depends on the
ventilation and on the fresh gas flow. The ventilation is most important in
the case of the V.I.C., but the fresh gas flow is most important with the
V.O.C. With regard to the V.O.C., the more you try to economize by reducing the fresh gas flow, less volume of vapour is added and the lower becomes the inhaled concentration. So that, if I can add to my colleague,
Dr. JOHNSTONE's, remark, I would say it is perfectly safe to use a closed circuit for halothane but only if you understand the influence of the three factors: the vaporizer concentration; the ventilation of the patient; and the fresh
gas flow. If you think of these three, you will quickly come to the conclusion,
which I came to a long time ago, that the only really safe method of using
a closed circuit with halothane is to put the Vaporizer Outside the Circuit.

Morris: Well, thank you very much. I think that I would like to use
that same slide for just a moment. That middle line which represents a
non-rebreathing circuit is the one which at least the beginner with a potent

anaesthetic agent could well afford to try for a while, even though the high flows of gases may be somewhat spendthrift, because there he can determine, within reasonable range and fairly accurately, the actual concentration which he is offering to the patient. To emphasize this in a little different way, I think that we need to see a slide that shows us something about vapour pressure curves. Dr. ARTUSIO, can you help here?

Artusio: Yes, I have some slides. The first one, Table 2, does not exactly show curves, but shows the saturated vapour pressures of several anaesthetics at 20° C, indicating the low saturated vapour pressure of methoxyflurane and the higher vapour pressures of drugs such as halothane, fluoroxene (Fluoromar), and diethyl ether. In addition to the saturated vapour pressures, the solubilities of these compounds in the aqueous and lipoid phases of the body will also determine in part their speed of induction and the speed of emergence from anaesthesia. The number of molecules per unit of time at any temperature that can be presented to the patient will be related to the saturated vapour pressure. The safety of vaporizers outside of the circuit has been mentioned but how can one be sure of the percentage of anaesthetic vapour the patient is receiving? To place complete faith in mechanical vaporizers, and forgetting that the thermostatic mechanism of the vaporizer may not be functioning, is fraught with danger. The dial reading may be greatly different from the concentration delivered to the patient.

Table 2. *Saturated vapour pressure at 20° C for halothane, fluoromar, penthrane, diethyl ether, and chloroform.*

The Saturated Vapour Pressure at 20° C of Several Anesthetic Agents

Methoxyflurane	25 mmHg
Chloroform	150 mmHg
Halothane	243 mmHg
Trifluroethylvinyl ether	300 mmHg
Diethyl ether	450 mmHg

I would like to stress the importance of attention to the physiological response of the patient for I believe that one should not be too confident with a vaporizer setting, even though it is placed outside of the circle. When you depend upon a mechanical device and do not primarily rely on the patient's physiological response, you are heading eventually for serious trouble.

The next slide of actual vapor pressure curves (Table 3), shows how temperature is related to saturated vapour pressure.

With an increase in temperature of any liquid, the saturated vapour pressure above that liquid will rise. It is important to notice that methoxyflurane (penthrane) would have to be raised to an extremely high temperature in order to achieve similar vapour pressures seen with diethyl ether,

 L. E. MORRIS

Table 3. *Comparative vapor pressure data: temperature, degrees centigrade at various pressures.*

Pressure (milli-meters of mercury)	760	400	200	100	40	20	10
Fluoromar (Trifluoro ethyl-vinyl ether)	43.2° C	27.0	+11.0	− 3.0	−	−	−
Fluothane (Halothane) (Trifluoro, mono-brom, mono-chlor, ethane)	50.2° C	32.8	16.1	+11.0	−18	−30	−41
Chloroform (Trichloro-methane)	61.3° C	42.7	24.4	+10.4	−7.1	−	−29.7
Penthrane (Methoxyflurane)	104.0° C	84.9	66.1	49.5	30.4	17.7	6.3

halothane, or fluoroxene. Although many feel that the penthrane induction time is rather slow because of its low saturated vapour pressure, heat should not be used to increase the speed of induction. Increasing the temperature of penthrane liquid would tend to negate the inherent anaesthetic safety of this agent.

In addition to the saturated vapour pressure, and the aqueous and lipoid solubility, the ability to respire the vapour will also determine the speed of anaesthetic induction. A drug like diethyl ether is quite irritating to the tracheobronchial tree and will slow induction time. Drugs like halothane or penthrane, which have minimal effects on the tracheobronchial tree, permit the patient to inhale higher concentrations. These physical factors: saturated vapour pressure, the irritability of the drug on the upper respiratory tract, and aqueous and lipoid solubility are physical parameters that will determine the time of uptake and distribution of the drug.

Morris: At this point I would like to ask the Members of the Panel to define potency of anaesthetic agents. What is it that makes a potent anaesthetic? Dr. HOLMDAHL?

Holmdahl: I would like first to stress the importance of the concepts just given by my Panel colleagues. These ideas are certainly known in the best centers and should be brought into the teaching in every anaesthetic department in the world. Then, to come back to potency, I would say that an agent which is very flexible, that is to say – that has very rapid induction – and will give a deep level of anaesthesia in a low concentration, is a potent anaesthetic agent.

Morris: Dr. Johnstohne, do you agree that potency is related to concentration?

Johnstone: Inevitably it must be related to the amount of the agent which we give. I have no doubt that if we could give a very large dose of ether – 30–40% quickly over a period of about half-a-minute – ether would be a potent anaesthetic. But obviously we could not give that concentration, because the patient would not take it. But, as a practical anaesthetist working with very fast-working surgeons, my only criterion of a potent anaesthetic agent is the induction. The quicker the induction, the more potent the anaesthetic.

Morris: Our pharmacology friends might define potency as something dealing with an M.L.D. 50, or with the ratio of anaesthetic effect over the likelihood of producing complete respiratory arrest. I wonder if we might not better define it here in accord with Dr. Artusio's earlier comments, and suggest that potency of an agent is related to the difference between its saturated vapour pressure and that vapour pressure which actually produces anaesthesia. Do you have a thought on that, Joe?

Artusio: Well, I think I would agree with what you have said. Certainly, when one thinks of the biologic potency of a molecule, one thinks in terms of concentration. But certainly it is also related to the structure of the molecule itself – because I have investigated per-halogenated methanes and per-halogenated ethanes which are convulsants rather than depressants. Now, once you achieve a molecular structure, with a certain angstrom distance between the molecules, you can develop depressants to the central nervous system. Now, you can make those molecules more potent in a biological sense by adding various atoms to the nucleus of the molecule. Depending upon what atoms are added to the nucleus of the molecule, boiling point will usually be raised and its potency increased (along with its toxicity). So, when one speaks of potency, he may mean many things. Potency has several facets. I think we have to consider the facet of molecular structure as well as the facet of concentration when we think of potency.

Morris: I would like to define it in a slightly different way. I think of potency, myself, as the time it takes to retrieve human error. With some anaesthetic agents we have more time than with other agents. In this sense, I think that perhaps chloroform is our most potent anaesthetic. And, in this sense, penthrane might be a more or less impotent agent.

Now, while Dr. Artusio had a slide about vapour pressure on the wall over there I, jotted down a few figures to use, because it has been my experience that many people just do not quite understand about vapour pressure. We all know about vapour dressure – but we think it is a little too complex to use. Therefore, let us go through the process of making our own vapour pressure curves on this rough chart I have here, in which the vertical axis is in millimeters of mercury pressure and the horizontal axis here is in degrees of centigrade. Now, let us think of water which we know has a boiling point of 100 degrees. That just means that the vapour pressure of water at that point is a saturated pressure of 760 mm of mercury, or one atmosphere. On the other hand, at freezing it is roughly down here at close to zero. A line between may give us an approximate vapour pressure curve for water. Now, let us try it with anaesthetic agents. Consider, first, chloroform, the boiling point of which is about 61° C., and the vapour pressure of chloroform at 25° is roughly a quarter of an atmosphere. Then we can join these two points and come out with a vapour pressure curve for chloroform. For methoxyflurane we have a boiling point of 104 and a vapour pressure at 20° of 23 mm of mercury, and so this lower one becomes the vapour pressure curve for methoxyflurane. Halothane boils at roughly 50°, while at 20° its saturated vapour pressure is roughly 0.3 of an atmosphere (240 mm of mercury), and so we can draw another line here to produce the vapour pressure curve for halothane. Similar curves can be made for ether, trilene, or any other liquids. Now, of what importance is this family of vapour pressure curves? Well, your operating room, or the conditions in which you give an anaesthetic, may not be 20° as Dr. Artusio's figures suggested. It may be 25°, and if you can extrapolate along your very rough vapour pressures' curves, you begin to see what a difference it actually makes in volume of vapour picked up at higher temperature when you must dilute that volume of saturated vapour with other anaesthetic gases, as we do in the Copper Kettle or Vernitrol types of apparatus.

Now, we are getting many more of your questions here, and I want to move on pretty fast. We have a question which has to deal with the relationship between relaxants and halothane. I wonder how many of the Panel actually feel it is necessary or desirable to use relaxants with halothane, and a corollary question is: Is there any contraindication between neostigmine and anaesthesia with fluothane? I would like to push that to you, Michael.

Johnstone: Well, I think that fluothane anaesthesia is possibly better with relaxants as regards abdominal surgery and thoracic surgery. If the dose of halothane is limited to the narcotic dose range, that is to say, between 30 and 40 ml, of vapour per minute in a closed system, vaporizer outside, I do not think it really matters what particular relaxant you use, whether it is a succinylcholine drip, flaxedil, or curare. Halothane, I think, either doubles or triples the sensitivity of the heart to prostigmine. The slowing effect from half a milligram of prostigmine in the conscious patient is doubled when the patient is anaesthetized. Therefore, we must be quite certain that we give a large dose of atropine to counteract the cardiac effects of prostigmine. One milligram is the usual, at the end of the operation.

Morris: Are there other ideas on this from any of the other Members?

Mushin: I would just like to translate Dr. JOHNSTONE's statement for the benefit of my clinical colleagues. If what he means is that a patient is being ventilated at anything between 8 and 10 liters a minute, and is inhaling about half to one percent, then I fully agree with all he says. His ideas are entirely accurate, but I still think it is easier for an anaesthetist to think of a patient being ventilated with 8 liters per minute of gas containing $^1/_2\%$ halothane than to talk of administration of 30 or 40 ml of theoretically pure halothane vapour. This is where the difficulty comes in. Thank you.

Johnstone: May I have the floor, Sir, for a moment? I think the failure to appreciate the difference between concentration and dosage of halothane has led to what is probably the biggest misunderstanding concerning halothane, particularly in the realm of obstetrics. Now, the vast majority of people believe that halothane is, as the World Health Organization and the Food and Drugs people say, primarily a uterine relaxant. Now, there is only one reason for this attitude, one group being responsible in 1958. It is because they did not appreciate the difference between concentration and dose. If I may illustrate with figures: In 1958, a group of workers demonstrated quite conclusively that halothane was a profound uterine relaxant. The method they used was a draw-over calibrated vaporizer set at 3% halothane. They did not measure the minute volume of the patients. The minute volume of the patient in labor, having pains, is anything up to 90 liters per minute – that, of course, is the outside limit. Let us say, at 20 liters on the average. These patients breathe this halothane 3% at a minute volume of 20 liters and therefore pick up 600 ml of halothane per minute. Even at 1%, and the same minute volume, it is 200 ml of halothane. That dose, of course, produces profound uterine paralysis.

Now, over the last couple of years, I have been measuring halothane effects on elective Cesarean sections, the ideal obstetric cases for the study of halothane, and I find that if I give one liter of oxygen, with 30 milliliters of vapour per minute, into a closed system of Waters – or any type of closed system – and oxygen only, that patient stays asleep. We get the relaxation with a relaxant and we have no bother whatsoever with the fetus or the uterus. And we have quite a nice, smoth anaesthesia. Therefore, I feel that this is the much more significant figure; and of course with high flows, supposing we use 10 liters to get that dose, which is the usual semi-open system, we would have to have a vaporizer which gives 0.3% and, with the possible exception of the Draeger, there is no vaporizer with that degree of accuracy at the low markings. Thank you.

Morris: I object to that last point. Certainly the Copper Kettle and the Vernitrol vaporizers provide discrete control of even greater accuracy over the entire range of concentrations, down to less than 0.3%. [Ref. FELDMAN, STANLEY A., & MORRIS, LUCIEN, E., *"Vaporization of halothane and ether in the copper kettle"*, Anaesthesiology **19**, 5, 650–655 (Sept-Oct) 1958.]

Mushin: Dr. JOHNSTONE and I are really in full agreement and the best proof of this is that we are prepared to discuss interpretation. If you have a flow of fresh gas of 1000 milliliters per minute of 3% halothane vapour (i.e., 30 milliliters per minute of halothane vapour) into a closed circuit, it must be quite obvious to everybody in this room that at least 700 milliliters of mixed gases escape into the outer air. It is quite impossible, therefore, for the patient actually to take 30 milliliters of halothane per minute into his body out of the fresh gas flow. I also spoke of ventilation of the patient's lungs, and this is the important measurement which the anaesthetist must make. Now, if we ventilate our patients' lungs with the necessary 10 liters per minute, and that contains 0.5% of halothane, it does not matter what vaporizer it comes out of, so long as you know that the concentration of halothane is 0.5%. With a ventilation of 10,000 milliliters, containing 0.5% halothane, 50 milliliters per minute halothane is in the patient's lungs which is the important place. Naturally, not all of it is absorbed. In fact, the uptake of halothane is of the order of 7–10 milliliters per minute with 0.5% halothane. I like to think always of ventilation and anaesthetic concentration in the trachea and then I arrive at, to me, a much more interesting figure. The milliliters per minute of halothane vapour entering the circuit or the patient's respiratory system is a nice theoretical figure to keep at the back of your mind (but it is a derived figure which is of probably little immediate practical importance). To my mind, ventilation and inspired concentration are the critical parameters which each one of us should know.

Morris: I would like to move on now to another topic. We have several questions dealing with arrhythmias. Dr. JOHNSTONE, do you think that we should be concerned about arrhythmias with the halogenated agents?

Johnstone: Arrhythmias are always significant of something, particularly the ventricular types. It is possible to give halothane in such a way – just adequate depth, efficient ventilation and removal of carbon dioxide – so that we do not see these arrhythmias. I think the ventricular arrhythmia usually is a reflection of the inadequate technique which is being used by the anaesthetist. And the other arrhythmias – the vagal types, the nodal rhythm, bradycardia – they indicate the need for a little bit of atropine perhaps, but they are always a significant warning and the anaesthetist should determine precisely what is causing them, at the time of their occurrence.

Morris: Do you recommend atropine to correct this difficulty?

Johnstone: Oh, no. Unless there is a reasonable clinical indication for it, I do not use atropine routinely. I use it if I am using a scoline drip because there one really sees the vagal disturbances during the halothane anaesthesia.

Morris: Let us change the frame of reference for just a moment, Dr. JOHNSTONE. I have a question in front of me here, wondering whether atropine should be used to antagonize the hypotension which is seen with halothane.

Johnstone: Well, it does tend to antagonize the hypotension, but I do not regard it as a good anti-hypotensive drug. I think that if one gets hypotension, one either reduces the dose of halothane or gets the blood volume up with the appropriate replacement solutions.

Morris: Very good. I strongly second your answer. I have another question here, dealing with irregularities and arrhythmias. It says, "What do you think about infiltration of the scalp with 20 to 40 cc. of a solution of adrenalin, 1:200,000, during the use of halothane?" Dr. MUSHIN?

Mushin: I am going to be provocative now, and say that in the present state of our knowledge, adrenalin should not be injected into a patient who is inhaling halothane. There have been a number of deaths which have been reported. In fact, two cardiac arrests occurred in my own teaching hospital. Fortunately, they were both resuscitated. These cardiac arrests in our own experience occurred shortly after the injection of adrenalin. There is ample pharmacological evidence that halothane, in common with some other halogenated anaesthetics, sensitizes the myocardium to the action of adrenalin, often to a very high degree. I would like to say rather firmly that adrenalin should not be used in conjunction with halothane in the present state of our knowledge.

Morris: That would apply equally well to trichlorethylene?

Mushin: Yes, that would apply equally well to trichlorethylene, and to chloroform.

Morris: I think it applies to chloroform, but perhaps not equally well. At least from our own experimental evidence, ventricular fibrillation is more easily demonstrated with trichlorethylene and perhaps with fluothane. It also appears to be less likely to occur during anaesthesia with fluoromar. I have another question along the same lines: Can adrenalin infiltration be used with penthrane, Dr. ARTUSIO?

Artusio: Some light can now be cast upon the sensitization of ventricular muscle produced by halogenated hydrocarbons. Our group studied a whole host of halogenated hydrocarbons and found both the spontaneously occurring ventricular irregularities, and the sensitization of the myocardium leading to an increased incidence of the ventricular irregularities produced by epinephrine always occurred with the administration of straight chain halogenated hydrocarbons. Those who use straight chain hydrocarbons in clinical anaesthesia must be warned against the simultaneous use of epinephrine. I do not believe that epinephrine should ever be used with straight chain halogenated hydrocarbon anaesthetics. I agree fully with Dr. Mushin that sometime you will get the right dose and the right concentration to produce serious ventricular irregularities. By the introduction of an ether-oxygen linkage into the straight chain hydrocarbon molecule, converting it to an ether, the occurrence of spontaneous ventricular beats is greatly decreased. The ether-oxygen bridge also decreases the ability of epinephrine to produce ventricular arrhythmias. However, even during an ether anaesthesia, the simultaneous use of epinephrine is still not safe. I would recommend to you that at no time are you absolutely safe using epinephrine with straight chain or ether linked hydrocarbon. This, of course, applies to penthrane as it is an ether hydrocarbon, but the incidence of the spontaneously occurring arrhythmias is much, much, less.

Morris: Your explanation also tends to support the lack of true sensitivity to epinephrine that we have seen with fluoromar, which is trifluoroethyl vinyl ether.

While discussing cardiac irregularities, we should consider another question here: does the advent of the beta receptor blockers alter the thinking about the use of epinephrine with several halogenated agents? In other words, could you prevent this response, Dr. Johnstone?

Johnstone: Yes, the whole picture is completely altered and there is every reason to believe that the beta receptor blocker interalia will be quite effective in cutting down the ventricular response to either endogenous or exogenous adrenalin. Now, I am quite happy about endogenous adrenalin. That is completely blocked. One can have a CO_2 retention if one wishes to practice anaesthesia that way. One can have very intense surgical stimulation and light planes of halothane. If the patient has a beta blocker, then there is absolutely no ventricular response to those noxious stimuli. It is going to be a problem, however, as to what can happen to the dose relationship between alderlin or inderal and exogenous catecholamines like adrenalin, because inderal at least is essentially a competitive blocker and therefore the amount of inderal required to block exogenous adrenalin will, of course, depend upon the amount of adrenalin administered and the route of administration. We have not embarked on that particular study as yet because, as I am sure you will understand, it is not a particularly attractive subject.

Holmdahl: I would like to come in here and ask Dr. JOHNSTONE how will the beta blockers affect the myocardial contractile force? It has been ample evidence that you have a sympathetic discharge, tonic discharge, the whole time to increase the myocardial contractile force, and if you block that sympathetic tonus – so to say, that sympathetic discharge – you will also decrease the myocardial contractile force. And I think we will come back soon how all these halogenated agents act on our vasomotor system, and I would like to ask you, how will these beta blockers affect the myocardial force together with halogenated agents?

Johnstone: Well, it will depend on the circumstances under which the blocker is administered. If the blocker is administered to a conscious patient who is not under stress – this is not my work; this has been done in London and it was with the predecessor drug, alderlin – there is no significant effect on the contractile force of the heart. Obviously this is a drug which is to suppress the stress reactions in the heart. If a person is not under catecholamine stress, it has no effect whatsoever. Now, as regards anaesthesia, if the patient is under catecholamine stress – that is to say, a very light plane of halothane anaesthesia, cyclopropane anaesthesia, or any type of anaesthesia which mobilizes catecholamines – and a surgical stimulus is applied, the blood pressure rises, the pulse rate rises, and one may even get extrasystoles quite frequently. When the alderlin is given at that stage, the contractile force of the heart is undoubtedly decreased, but it simply is brought back to normal.

Holmdahl: May I interrupt here a little bit? My point was that you have the basic sympathetic discharge to the heart the whole time, and it has been shown lately by RUSSEL in Stockholm, and the FONTGO group in Göteborg, that if you block the sympathetic system you also decrease in a basic state the myocardial contractive force.

Johnstone: I was speaking about conscious subjects, rather than unconscious, anaesthetized subjects.

Holmdahl: We can speak first about the conscious subjects. There you decrease the myocardial contractile force, and I think that you will decrease it to the same degree providing the halogenated agent has not already taken away all sympathetic discharge to the heart. But we do not use the halogenated agents in this concentration.

Johnstone: As I said before, it depends on the circumstances. Here we have a slide (Fig. 5) that shows ventricular arrhythmias altered by or influenced by Inderal. On the top two tracings, top left is a ventricular arrhythmia during very light halothane anaesthesia, with intense surgical stimulation, sudden opening of the knee joint. To the right of that tracing is the peripheral pulse, a plethysmograph type of tracing which we think indicates the contractile force and the stroke volume of the heart. Notice how the pulse is most erratic, some beats extremely weak. We gave the blocker and forty seconds later we have a normal sinus rhythm and a stroke volume which is incomparably better.

Drugs	Electrocardiogram Lead 2	Digital pulse wave Recorder sensitivity 0,5 mv /0,5 cm	B.P. Systolic
Atropine 1,0 mg. Halothane, light Surgical stimulation +++ of knee joint Robust male 32 yr. Spontaneous resp.			90 mm, Hg.
30 secs. after Pronethalol 15 mg. intravenously Spontaneous resp.			120 mm, Hg.

Fig. 5. Ventricular arrhythmias corrected by Inderal cf. Fig. 4, Brit. J. Anaesthesia **36**: 228, 1964 – Reproduced by permission.

Morris: Thank you. May we have the lights again? We will go on, then, to other somewhat related topics. I have several questions here dealing with hypotension, and am wondering whether Dr. ARTUSIO would like to explain the cause of the hypotension with Penthrane. Is this a lower cardiac output, or vasodilation, or is it a ganglionic blocking effect?

Artusio: I wish I knew the answer to that question. When a vagotonic drug like halothane is used, some of the fall in blood pressure can be associated with cardiac slowing. The use of atropine, under these circumstances, will raise the blood pressure as the heart increases its rate. However, as you know, with the halogenated anaesthetics, atropine raises the blood pressure only occasionally, and when it does, the fall in blood pressure was related to cardiac slowing. Therefore, I believe that with increase in concentration, all of the halogenated anaesthetics in common use today, lower the blood pressure by direct myocardial depression and with only a minimal amount of peripheral dilatation. As for ganglionic blocking action, the evidence is not complete. There is some data to indicate that halothane and penthrane have ganglionic blocking properties and others do not. In view of the available data, I think that it behooves us to use the halogenated anaesthetics in the lightest level compatible with the surgical procedure, and that one should at all times attempt to have a patient's blood pressure as high as possible during adequate surgical operating conditions. I know that today most of us tolerate a lower blood pressure than we would with drugs like diethyl ether and cyclopropane and some would indicate to us that this lower blood pressure is satisfactory, that we need not worry about a low blood pressure with fluothane or penthrane. I think that there is some truth to that. However, in spite of our belief that one can have a lower blood pressure, one should not forget our old practices of maintaining the status quo as nearly as possible. I fully believe that the main portion of the fall in blood pressure, associated with halogenated anaesthetics, is related to direct myocardial depression.

Morris: Is there someone on the Panel who should like to add or take exception to that?

Johnstone: Yes, as far as halothane is concerned, this term "myocardial depression" is meaningless because nobody has ever proved that one way or the other. The most interesting work done has been at Philadelphia by the Dripps group, in which they show that if halothane got into the brain with a separate circulation, all the peripheral effects were produced. Therefore, the only reasonable conclusion that we can draw from that particular experiment is that halothane depresses the blood pressure, slows the heart, etc., by blocking the sympathetic nervous system. And if we block the sympathetic nervous system, as we know from total spinal , the cardiac output drops precipitously, eventually to zero sometimes. Now, in the intact human subject or the intact animal, it is impossible to dissociate the sympathetic innervation, the Purkinje fibers, the sympathetic nerve fibers, etc., from the myocardial cells. Therefore, it is illogical to state that any anaesthetic that we know at the present time is a myocardial depressant. Cardiac depressant, yes, direct or indirect. But fluothane appears to be an indirect depressant, and if I might show you tracings of digital plethysmography, it will undoubtedly show the dilatation of the peripheral vessels, which is quite sufficient to account for the blood pressure changes.

Now, these are digital pulse waves taken from a single patient (Fig. 6). Reading from the top, the time on the far left, the halothane dose next, then the pulse waves, followed by blood pressure and a few remarks. Notice that once we get the patient deeply anaesthetized, at minute seven, we have considerable peripheral vasodilatation, but not a lot of drop in blood pressure, 140 to 100, which simply the abolition of consciousness in an acutely apprehensive patient would account for. If we push the halothane there is a considerable further drop in blood pressure, without any tendency to vasoconstriction. The drop in blood pressure is smartly reversed by the withdrawing of the drug. I think that is proof positive of peripheral vasodilatation accounting for drops in blood pressure.

Time in minutes	Halothane dose MI vapour per minute	Pulse wave Recorder sensitivity imv/icm Standard ECG speed 2.5 cm/sec	Systolic blood pressure mm Hg (digital)	Remarks
0	0	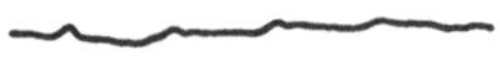	140	Conscious & apprehensive
2	0	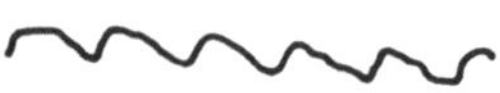	120	Thiopentone 200 mg. Asleep Spontaneous resp^{tn}
7	300	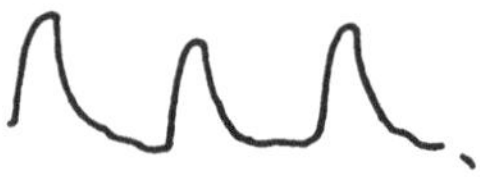	100	Spontaneous respiration Endotracheal anaesthesia
30	60	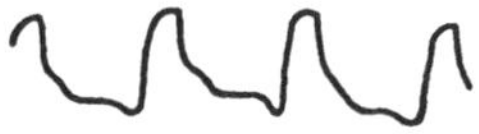	95	Dura tense, Spontaneous respiration
60	60	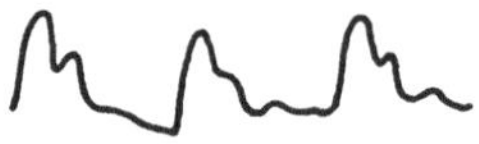	70	Controlled respiration. Aneurysm visible
64	100	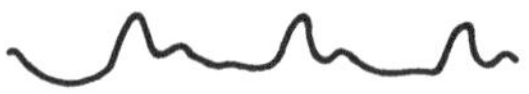	40	Controlled respiration
70	0	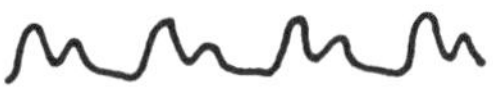	40	Controlled respiration Aneurysm clipped
80	40	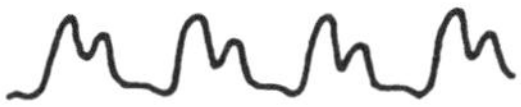	85	Spontaneous respiration
130	0	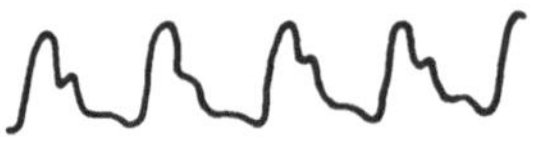	100	Operation complete

Fig. 6. Digital pulse waves relating peripheral vasodilatation to blood pressure drop from halothane. Reproduced by Permission from Johnstone, M.; Halothane: The First Five Years. Anes. **22**: 591, 1961.

Holmdahl: I would like to come back here to agree with Dr. JOHN-STONE that halothane certainly is a sympathetic blocker. And it has been evidently shown now that not only do you have a basic sympathetic discharge giving a certain myocardial contractile force, but you also have a sympathetic discharge the whole time to control your peripheral vascular resistance. And if you know about sympathetic discharge, you will also have a peripheral vascular dilatation at the same time as you have a lowering of the myocardial contractile force, and I think we only speak about differences in concentration of the sympathetic blocking agent. And there I just want to point out that while we do not see this with, for example, old good ether, it is because we have at the same time an increased sympathetic discharge with ether. Ether, as all other anaesthetic agents, is a myocardial depressing agent, but you have an increased sympathetic discharge compensating for this, and I think one here really ought to bring out the point that you must know what is the state of your patient: is he able to have his intact homeostatic vasomotor regulatory mechanism?

Mushin: I agree with Dr. JOHNSTONE. We cannot be too precise about the exact site of action of fluothane. I am sure Dr. HOLMDAHL is correct that it is partly sympathetic blockade. But at any rate, from the clinician's point of view, the blood pressure fall should be interpreted as being due to a falling cardiac output as the major cause. The remarkable thing about the cardiac output under fluothane is that it is so sensitive to dosage. Now, this has not been confirmed in human beings directly because it is so difficult to get serial cardiac output measurements. PAYNE has attempted this. But it has been shown in animal experiments. In the article on halothane in the British Medical Journal in 1956 by the Medical Research Council team, you will find the graph showing the effect of different concentrations of fluothane on cardiac output. As clinicians, we know how easy it is to raise the blood pressure by reducing the concentration of halothane. I feel it is cardiac output which is the main factor concerned.

Holmdahl: I would like to come in here because you often see anaesthetic techniques advocated to push fluothane to use, let us say, the good effects of hypotension. And I would like to bring to you the concept of oxygen transport nicely put out by JOHN NUNN, in England. I think this is so important that every anaesthetist should be aware that the oxygen transport – that is to say, the flux of oxygen over the aortic valve – is determined by the three basic things: cardiac output; times the hemoglobin you have – that is to say, the oxygen carrying capacity; – times your saturation. Normally, in adult man, you have 5,000 milliliters of blood per minute going over the aortic valve. You have, in a non-anemic patient, 20 milliliters of oxygen in 100 milliliters of blood and, as anaesthetists, you should always see, too, that he has 100% saturation. That is to say, that the oxygen flux, the available oxygen for the patient, is 1,000 milliliters per minute. If you have an oxygen consumption of, let us say, 200–250 milliliters, we can say per-minute, that will give us an extraction so that you will have a venous oxygen saturation level of 75%. Now, a man normally very easily compensates for a decrease in oxygen carrying capacity, or even a decrease in saturation, by increasing the cardiac output. But now we have discussed for a moment or two about the effects of different halogenated agents and we have all agreed that pushed to a higher level, you will have a decrease in cardiac output. If we then get a decrease in cardiac output, for example, just a one-third reduction in cardiac output, that will leave two-thirds of the oxygen transport here. If you have also an anemic patient with reduction down to 13 milliliters for 100 milliliters of blood, that will leave you two-thirds normal. And you may also get a decrease of oxygen saturation. Let us say that each of these factors is reduced to two-thirds. You have, as a matter of fact, $2 \times 2 \times 2$, that will be 8 over $3 \times 3 \times 3$; that is 8/27 of your available oxygen, and this is a quite impossible situation for this patient, because now he has not more than 300 milliliters, or something like that, of available oxygen, and he must extract everything and lower his oxygen tension in the tissue. So, whenever you use high levels of anaesthetic agents, with a reduction in cardiac output, you certainly must see too that you have a 100% saturation of your hemoglobin and you must see, too, that you do not have a bleeding because a hypovolemic situation will also harm circulation more than anaemia. And now, I would like to stress this—that this is not so easy as you think, to get a 100% saturation, for example, in a bled patient. There is ample evidence, firstly, I think, put out by DURST, RATTENBORG and HOLADAY in the States, FREEMAN and NUNN from England, and now I have just seen some data by KAI REHDER that, in a bled patient, due to alteration of the ventilation perfusion ratios, you always have an increase in the functional dead space. And to compensate for that, you have to hyperventilate the patient. So, under these circumstances, it may be very wise to increase the oxygen tension in the inspired mixture. In most instances, God's good air may be right. But, under clinical anaesthesia, in a bled patient, with difficulties in keeping an airway free or keeping up alveolar ventilation, you certainly will use a little bit of extra oxygen.

Morris: Thank you very much, Dr. HOLMDAHL, for this excellent graphic demonstration of why we need to give our patients the best. We will change now and go on to something else then for a little bit. I would like to ask all Members of the Panel in minimal words: Is halothane an analgesic?

Mushin: I do not see how any anaesthetic can fail to be an analgesic in sub-anaesthetic doses. It is all part of the same process and I am unable to understand what my colleagues mean when they speak of analgesia due to a drug which is an anaesthetic when given in sufficient dosage, but when given in lesser doses produces a state of blurring of the sensorium. This is called, quite incorrectly of course, analgesia. It is not analgesia, but half-anaesthesia. And I think any anaesthetic given in sub-anaesthetic doses will produce this state of half-anaesthesia.

Holmdahl: I think that there is ample evidence that trichlorethylene and Penthrane have a more analgetic potential in a less depressed central nervous system range than fluothane.

Johnstone: I think the term "analgesia" is being abused at the present time to fit in with certain rather nebulous theories. Halothane was synthesized and developed as a general anaesthetic. It has got absolutely nothing to do with analgesia. Analgesia being defined as a loss of pain perception without interference with consciousness. The only example we have of it, of course, is local analgesia, or spinal.

Artusio: Well, this of course is a very interesting question and it depends a great deal on semantics. However, I think that perhaps there are very few true analgetics in the pure sense of the term.

Diethylether is the classical anaesthetic. It indeed produces a rise in pain threshold, before the loss of consciousness. I have some reasons to believe, however – and this is purely hypothesis on my part – and you will take it or leave it, as you will – that the series of halogenated compounds are not true analgetics, but behave more like the vast group of sedatives and hypnotics. The onset of analgesia follows the loss of consciousness, as with the sedative and hypnotic drugs. The recoveries from anaesthesia are associated with muscle fasciculation so often seen during recovery from sedative and hypnotic anaesthesia. For these reasons, I would question a good deal the true analgesic nature of the halogenated anaesthetics. If a drug like pentothal is an analgetic when one pushes it to very deep hypnotic levels in which the patient does not respond to the surgical stimulus, then I think the halogenated anaesthetics are analgesics. But I agree that in the purest sense of the word an analgesic is a drug that raises the pain threshold without the loss of consciousness.

Morris: Dr. MUSHIN, do you care to reply to that?

Mushin: I am completely at loss after hearing that. Just what is an anaesthetic? I agree with my colleague, Dr. JOHNSTONE, that the only true analgesics we have are the local analgesics. All analgesic drugs given systemically produce a range of depression of pain sensitivity, but always with a range of depression of the general sensorium – that is the general level of consciousness. I would like to hear of one which, injected systemically, raises pain threshold without at the same time altering, in some degree, the general sensory level.

Johnstone: I think we are getting fairly close to that with the phenoperidines . . .

Mushin: I am sorry to show some surprise at this. Are you implying that injection of any of the peridines, whether it is meperidine, phenoperidine, haloperidine or droperidine, raises the pain threshold without altering the general level of sensory activity? There is not one individual in this whole room who, if given the smallest dose of these peridines, would not have a generalized sensory depression, whatever happened to his pain threshold.

Johnstone: Yes, that is probably correct. I simply said that perhaps we are getting a bit closer to the definition of analgesia.

Morris: You will agree, however, that either some sort of hoax has been perpetrated in the past, or that trichlorethylene and chloroform at least, and perhaps more recently penthrane, do have some effects in at least minimal anaesthetic levels which some of these other anaesthetic agents do not have.

Johnstone: I have been looking at this recently in obstetrics and, as far as I can make out, all these agents act similarly; that is, the inhalation agents from nitrous onwards. The only description I can give to the change which occurs in the patient is that the patient's attitude toward the pain is altered, but the pain perception does not appear to be changed significantly.

Morris: This fits in with an old concept of mine, dealing with the effect of muscle relaxants, which perhaps is pertinent to this discussion. I believe that anything which alters the total afferent input may alter the ability to interpret a stimulation as pain and therefore removes the need for analgesics. Perhaps this is the way anaesthetics work in less than anaesthetic concentrations.

Mushin: Well, I would suggest for a start, Mr. Chairman, that we give up the term analgesic or analgesia when we are considering drugs given directly into the blood stream or by inhalation. In other words, we ought not to speak of systemically administered drugs as being analgesics. Let us talk of half anaesthesia, or partial anaesthesia, and then we will know what we mean. Now, I have taken part in many series of experiments concerning analgesia and, if my colleague Sir ROBERT MACINTOSH is here, he will recall many of them because he was with me. Varying concentrations of inhalation anaesthetics were administered and the subjects, all trained doctors, not only recorded their own observations, but also had many observations made on them. I can assure you that, in the case certainly of ether, trichlorethylene, chloroform, and ethylchloride (I have not done this with halothane yet), it is not so much the appreciation of the character of the pain which is altered, nor the intensity, but it is the motor response to the pain which is altered, right up to the moment of complete unconsciousness.

Morris: I think we need to move on to other aspects now. I have here a question which deals with the asthmatic patient. What about halogenated anaesthetics in the asthmatic patient? Is there a special reason to use halogenated anaesthetics and, if so, which one? Dr. ARTUSIO?

Artusio: I think as far as anaesthetic agents in the asthmatic patient, diethylether appears to be the choice in our institution. We have used penthrane very successfully in the asthmatic patients, relieving the asthma. It might be a common quality of most of the anaesthetics. I would prefer the ether type of compound.

Johnstone: Well, I have not used anything else except halothane, and it seems to be perfectly satisfactory and, in the area in which I live, we have a lot of these bronchospastic conditions due to the pollution of the air.

Holmdahl: We do not have so much of these bronchospastic diseases as in England; we do not have that same air pollution, but lately we have seen quite a lot of severe status asthmatics coming in. It may have something to do with widespread use of corticosteroids. I will not go into this discussion now and I get out of it by getting to the status asthmaticus. And we prefer, perhaps, to use halothane over ether to get rid a little bit of the sticky secretion. But I think the most important thing – and I come back to my oxygen transport concept – is to support ventilation, correct acid-base status, and make them responsive again to adrenergic drugs. If you can correct the acid-base status, they will be dilated by adrenergic drugs and we there have one of the few indications, I would say, for use of Tris (hydroxymethyl aminomethane), the THAM drug, because that will correct the intracellular acidosis.

Morris: I have another brief question: What influence does penthrane have on blood coagulation?

Artusio: None at all.

Morris: Another question that gets back to an earlier discussion: Is there any elapsed time which should be allowed to go by as far as epinephrine and halothane, or epinephrine with any of the other anaesthetics? Would it be safe, for instance, to inject epinephrine, 1/200,000, and then give halothane half an hour later?

Mushin: Well, I think this is rather a matter of guess work. Giving epinephrine and then halothane half an hour later would, I think, be all right because, judging by its blood pressure effects at any rate, the effect of epinephrine would have disappeared by then.

Morris: Judging by the charts that we saw here in another panel two or three days ago, it continues on as far as demonstrable blood levels are concerned, for a considerable length of time – longer than thirty minutes.

Mushin: Epinephrine?

Morris: Yes.

Mushin: Well, I think it is much better to observe the rule. Just do not give epinephrine at all into a patient to whom you propose to give halothane.

Holmdahl: Are we still discussing the use of epinephrine together with halothane in status asthmaticus? Then I just would like to bring up the point that if you have to use epinephrine in this situation, you just use it, because again I would like to stress the oxygen transport situation. You have to improve that. And I would even take the risk, to use adrenalin together with halothane in such a situation. And there is another thing with that, too; we should never forget that in a deranged acid-base status, the patient is very much less sensitive to epinephrine than in a normal acid-base status.

Mushin: I entirely agree with the need to treat a patient suffering from an asthmatic attack with adrenalin if necessary, but why pick on fluothane when we have many other anaesthetics?

Artusio: I would like to say that I think that, with any anaesthetic used, intubation of the patient and clearing the tracheobronchial tree of secretions might help eliminate the acid-base balance problem more than the use of epinephrine in trying to dilate the bronchi. I think that once the secretions are removed, a very prompt response of the patient occurs, associated certainly with surgical ether anaesthesia.

Holmdahl: I think this has nothing perhaps to do any longer with the clinical use of halogenated agents, but I just would like to say that still patients are dying from status asthmaticus – and more and more in many countries. And if we intubate, and even if we try to suck out, it may be very, very difficult to dilate the bronchus enough to have enough oxygenation of that patient.

Morris: I think I would like to get us back to the question. I think the difficulty arises in the minds of a good many anaesthetists when they have committed themselves already to fluothane anesthesia, and when the surgeon, comes along and announces he is going to infiltrate this or that part of the anatomy with some vasoconstrictor, I think that we can nicely solve the problem by educating the surgeon to use another agent, such as neosynephrine, for instance. Most of the surgeons that we have tried to educate in this direction seem to be quite well pleased.

I have a further question here: What are the toxic products of fluothane in respect to rubber and its contact with and solution in rubber? Is anyone on the Panel prepared to talk about that? Dr. MUSHIN?

Mushin: I do not know the chemistry of this, but I certainly know that fluothane is taken up by rubber. If any of you propose undertaking any analytical studies of fluothane concentration, be careful what kind of tubing is used to convey the mixture from one place to another, because if you use rubber your results may not be valid.

Morris: Anyone want to comment about any toxic product with rubber? ... The Panel apparently knows of none at this point.

Holmdahl: May be we ought to discuss a little bit what evidence we have for the metabolic degradation of fluothane and other halogenated agents in the body.

Morris: I was actually going to come to that. To do so, may be we ought to first go back to our oldest halogenated agent. Dr. ARTUSIO, will you tell us something about chloroform metabolism?

Artusio: Some years ago, Dr. VAN POZNAK and I, and Dr. BELLVILLE, working with servomechanisms, found that during cyclopropane anaesthesia a rather constant amount of cyclopropane would have to be added to the system during the steady state. At that time, this was thought to be due to loss of gas through the rubber parts of the system. This loss bothered us and for several years we wondered whether there could be a bio-transformation of the so-called inert anaesthetic agents. Eventually, Dr. VAN POZNAK was able to get some C-14 labeled $CHCl_3$, and he and Dr. CHENOWETH, at the Dow Chemical Company, performed some experiments on the rat and found that C-14 carbon dioxide could be collected as an end-product.

This meant that there was bio-transformation (Fig. 7) of chloroform in the organism and that chloroform was not truly inert. There are some other data now that would indicate that most of the anaesthetic agents that we use today undergo some bio-transformation in the organism and are not inert.

This means, then, that all the computer systems that are programmed to study uptake and distribution now have to take into consideration a certain amount of biotransformation in the organism. Whether this amount of biotransformation has anything to do with toxicitiy of anaesthetic agents, we do not know. We have no idea what the intermediary products of this biotransformation are. We know only that C-14 labeled carbon dioxide can be collected in these experiments, on the rat.

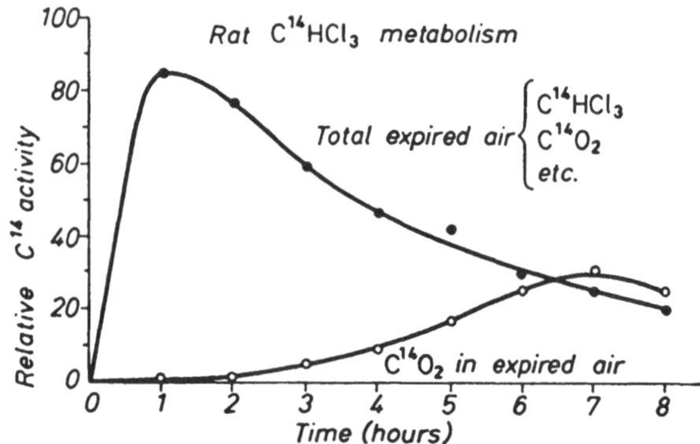

Fig. 7. Metabolism of Volatile Anaesthetics: Conversion in Vivo of Several Anaesthetics to Carbon Dioxide and Chloride. BioChem. Pharmacology **13**: 1239–1247, 1964. Van Dyke, Chenoweth, Van Poznak, Pergamon Press, Ltd.

Morris: Will you tell us about trichlorethylene, Dr. Mushin?

Mushin: I am sure you all know that a good deal of the trichlorethylene which is inhaled is broken down to trichloro-acetic acid which is excreted by the kidneys. Fig. 8, also computed by Mapleson, is most fascinating. It shows the relationship between the time taken for the arterial blood to come into equilibrium with inhaled concentrations of different anaesthetics. Now, in the case of cyclopropane and of nitrous oxide, you see equilibrium has occurred rapidly. Arterial blood and inhaled concentration are almost at the same level, at the end of about one hour. At the end of ten minutes, 80% equilibrium has already occurred. In the case of halothane, 80% equilibrium does not occur for anything up to 24 hours of administration. But, with trichlorethylene it looks as though equilibrium will never occur. The low horizontal nature of the trichlorethylene curve is due to a constant drain from the blood stream of trichlorethylene by conversion into trichloro-acetic acid, amongst other things, which is excreted by the kidneys. All the other anaesthetics do eventually come into equilibrium if they are administered for long enough. In the case of methoxyflurane, you must administer it for about five weeks in order to get something like 80% equilibrium between arterial blood and inhaled concentration. It has been confirmed by many workers that trichlorethylene is broken down into trichloro-acetic acid. From my knowledge of experiments done over twenty years ago, the excretion of trichloro-acetic acid after a single administration of trichlorethylene lasting about one hour, goes on for nearly two weeks. And many patients, even after leaving the hospital, are still excreting trichloro-acetic acid. This is at least partly due to the build up of trichlorethylene which occurs in the fat reservoirs.

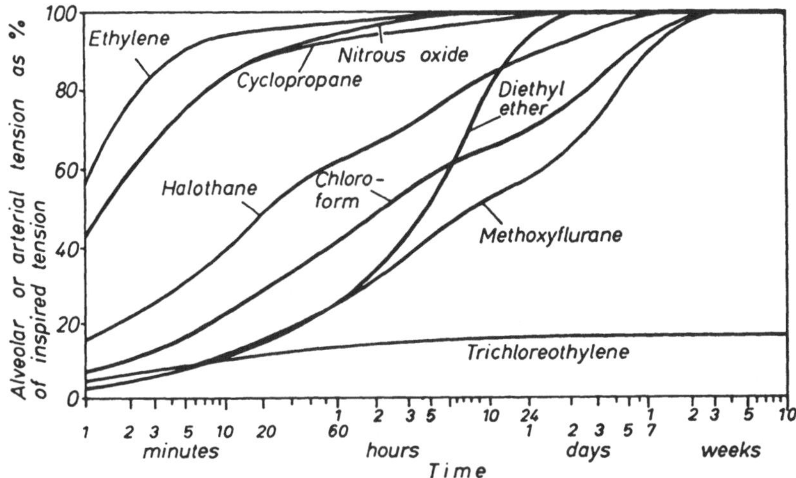

Fig. 8. Time taken for arterial blood to equilibrate with different anaesthetic concentrations.
Mapleson, W. W. (1963) in Papper and Kitz, "Uptake and Distribution of Anaesthetic Agents"

Morris: I think that there is some data which is accumulating from good work that indicates there is some metabolic breakdown of halothane as well and, from Dr. MUSHIN's remarks, it would seem that perhaps we ought to re-evaluate a number of these anaesthetics.

I had reserved the last half hour of our comments for some discussion of the liver problem with the various halogenated anaesthetics and I am going to lead into it by asking about pediatric anaesthesia. I would like each Member of the Panel to tell me whether he has any reservations about giving fluothane anaesthesia to children and, if so, at what age. Quickly, Dr. MUSHIN.

Mushin: I have no reservations about giving fluothane to children.

Morris: Dr. HOLMDAHL?

Holmdahl: No, I have no reservations in any age to give fluothane if needed.

Morris: Dr. JOHNSTOHNE?

Johnstone: No reservations.

Morris: Dr. Artusio?

Artusio: No reservations.

Morris: All right. Now then, do you feel, as a group, that it is safe to use Fluothane or halothane in the presence of liver disease?

Artusio: I would avoid the use of any halogenated anaesthetics in the presence of known liver disease.

Morris: Why?

Artusio: Because I believe that the halogenated anesthetics are associated with some degree of liver cell irritation, which is not significant in patients with a normal liver, which is the reason that none of us had qualms about giving it to the young liver.

Morris: It should be remembered also that there is a marked species difference in response of altered liver function after exposure to halogenated anaesthetics. There is a difference, too, in effect between halogenated agents. Fluoromar, in our clinical studies, has not been followed by any significant alterations in liver function after carbon dioxide stress similar to that which has produced changes when applied during chloroform, halothane, and methoxyflurane anaesthesia.

Johnstone: I have no reservations at all giving halothane anaesthetics to patients with liver disease, and constantly do so. I think the acid test of liver disease, of course, is portocaval anastomosis. I think it was last Monday that quite a fascinating paper by Dr. Havers showed that there is no significant difference between liver function after this operation under halothane or after epidural block.

Holmdahl: We have not had any contraindication so far, but we are certainly anxiously looking out for data from prospective studies. Now, we had a retrospective study by Dr. Mushin here, and he certainly will perhaps tell you a little bit about his data, but I think that the retrospective studies so far did not give us too much worry to use it if needed. On the other hand, in clearcut liver diesease it would be wise not to use halothane until we have these prospective studies done in a big group of patients. I know they are doing it in the States and I hope that they will do it in Dr. Mushin's and other United Kingdom departments, or any other departments where you can collect a big, well-controlled amount of material.

Morris: At that point I think I should tell this group that the studies in the States are as yet just finishing the retrospective phase. The National Research Council Committee has not yet released the information on the retrospective phase, but I would expect that it is very similar to that which has been done by several individuals and institutions, and very similar to that which has been done and reported by Dr. MUSHIN. Could you take two minutes and tell us a little something about that?

Mushin: I would have answered your question, Mr. Chairman, by saying that no anaesthetic at all ought to be administered to a patient with a damaged liver. The main point which emerged from my own studies was that all the common anaesthetics produce some degree of liver disturbance. But halothane did not produce any more liver disturbance than the others. This was true for all age groups, all durations of anaesthesia, all different sites of operation, and so on. This was shown not only by the results of liver function tests, but it was also shown by a very important observation (important in Great Britain, at any rate) of the duration of stay of the patient in hospital. Because we have used this observation on many other occasions, we know it is a very sensitive indicator of postoperative complications. The reasons for that you may guess at, but this is not the place to explain why it is so. All we can say at the moment is that there is no evidence, from our own studies and of others, that fluothane produces any more or any different kinds of liver disturbance than the other anaesthetics.

Holmdahl: I think it would be only fair to mention – as I come from a country where we use halothane quite a lot and we have not done, in most of the centers, any retrospective studies – we do not see what we do not look out for, and many of us have not looked back. But Dr. LÖFSTRÖM, at Serafimerlasarettet, has looked back in 13,000 anaesthetics given during the years 1959 to 1962. He has, during this period, 6,000 with halothane alone. He has another group of ether, about 3,500, and local anaesthetics 3,500. (We had one thing which is good for a retrospective study: nearly 100% of the patients dying in a Swedish hospital go to dissection.) And he has, in several of these section cases, histopathologically demonstrated necrosis of liver cells. All were in the halothane group. He has had two cases of severe liver damage after minor surgery, both in the halothane group. Again I think it is very difficult to get back to anaesthetic charts and be sure what the blood pressure level has been, and so on. Again I would like to stress here that we do not have enough evidence to blame halothane specially for this, and deduct so many other advantages. But we certainly must have well controlled prospective studies set up now.

Morris: Will anyone add to that?

Johnstone: Yes, Sir. I should think that the basic cause of the present controversy regarding the liver and halothane has its basis, purely and simply, in the fact that those responsible for precipitating it did not look back far enough. This is not a new syndrome. It has been thoroughly documented over the last twenty-five years, at least. The rather sad tale started in 1937 and perhaps – maybe later – I should run down briefly the history from 1937 till 1964, and show quite easily that this is not a new syndrome.

Morris: Michael, may I interrupt just a moment and tell the audience that, if they look back far enough, they will see that acute yellow atrophy was first described by Rokitansky in 1842, five years before the introduction of chloroform. Now, go ahead and make us up-to-date.

Johnstone: Yes. Well, it rather looks as though those who were responsible in some places far away, were perhaps living in an underdeveloped area as regards library facilities. Now, 1937 actually is a reasonable time to start. That year saw the first report of jaundice after pentothal, which was written up by a physician who did not give the anaesthetic, as toxic liver jaundice following pentothal. During the war years, it was discovered that virtually any parenteral injection could be followed by jaundice, which was occasionally fatal, from liver necrosis. The minimal incubation period, established at that time by the innoculation of volunteers, was sixteen days. After the war, several excellent studies were published, describing the pathology of shock. Liver necrosis featured very prominently in patients where there were medical illnesses, war wounds, etc.; patients who died with the blood pressure in its lower levels for twelve hours prior to death frequently showed liver necrosis. Similarly, after the war, we had postoperative jaundice attributed to penicillin and sulfonamides. Now there is reasonable evidence to indicate that both these drugs produce a true allergy and it is a comparatively easy experiment to cause liver necrosis by the antigen-antibody reaction in a sensitized liver. We know the incidence of penicillin allergy. Around about 1952, in the New England Journal – which also carried the halothane stories – we have 30 cases of postoperative jaundice attributed to postoperative aureomycin. Very recently, two years ago during the time of the halothane furor, we had 41 cases of jaundice following an intravenous barbiturate. Fifteen of these patients died from liver necrosis. The cause was traced to the use of multi-dose containers for the drug. Multi-dose containers are used and issued in many hospitals, to my knowledge, still. I think we should come to the conclusion very smartly everywhere that the hollow needle and the multi-dose container for drugs cannot be maintained in a proper state of sterility as regards virus. Thus we have three obvious causes for postoperative jaundice which have not been considered in any of the cases attributed to halothane. We have the reaction to trauma – shock by vasoconstriction in the liver. We have the transmission of virus, and we have the possibility of coincidental virus hepatitis. And finally we have the so-called allergic reactions to drugs, drugs in the antibiotic, tranquilizer, anticoagulant, a tremendously long list of them. None of them have received proper consideration in the analysis of the halothane cases.

Artusio: I would agree with everything that has been said. However I think, until the issue is clear, that rather than incriminate these anaesthetic agents, it is better not to use them in the presence of liver disease.

Johnstone: There is one point there, Sir, which I think it is right at the foundations of anaesthesia as a specialty. Anaesthetists are entitled to the same ethical considerations as their colleagues in other specialties. I draw your attention to one particular paper, published by LINDENBAUM and LEIFER in the New England Journal of Medicine. These two persons are physicians. They have no connection with surgery, no connection with anaesthesia. By some means which they did not disclose, they obtained the records of a department of anaesthetics, they collected nine cases, they published these cases without acknowledging permission from either the anaesthetists or the surgeons. Now, as far as I am concerned, that seems to be a rather disturbing departure from the accepted code of behaviour on the part of professional men, particularly in medicine. And therefore I am particularly surprised that the editor of that particular journal accepted the information obtained in that peculiar manner. I mentioned that case in particular because practically every factor which I mentioned earlier in relation to liver reactions was included in those eight to nine cases. But not a single reference to the fact that those factors had previously been held responsible, also in that particular journal.

Mushin: Could I just refer to one point which I mentioned in my paper yesterday and which, from discussion with members in the Congress, I did not make quite clear. And since many of you may be embarking on retrospective studies – and I hope many of you will – this may save you a good deal of effort and possibly even error. Now, of the many things which you will study in any retrospective investigation of this topic, one of them is almost certain to be results of liver function tests. There is a large number of these tests. But, without exception, the normal value – this is the word used – is always given as a range. In many instances, the range may be from one to ten. The difficulty always is to decide whether a particular liver function result is "normal" or "abnormal". Supposing the range given is one to ten, and your patient has a preoperative or an immediate postoperative result of 2 units. Now, is this normal or, if it goes from 2 to 8, is he still normal or has his liver got worse? This is the difficulty we found ourselves in and no one could give us the answer until we thought this out for ourselves. Now it became clear that this range of values, in reality, represented the distribution of values that you find in a normal population. We wrote to the authors who first described the individual liver function tests and asked for the experimental results on which the first description in the medical literature was based. With a single exception, – the test dealing with thymol turbidity –, we were given these original data. We were able to plot, perhaps for the first time, the distribution curve of values of liver function tests in normal populations. In general, they have the usual distribution curve of a natural biological phenomenon, and it was when we had plotted these natural distributions that we were then able to compare them with our own results. I do not think that any clear answer will ever come from studies of individual cases, as was suggested by Dr. HOLMDAHL, because in any individual case there will always be a large number of factors evolving around the patient's disease, the operation, the anaesthetic, and so forth. One must compare the distribution of values in a normal, healthy population, with a distribution of values of each liver function test in halothane patients, and compare that with non-halothane patients, and then calculate whether the difference between halothane and non- halothane, in large numbers of patients, is significant or not. This is what we did, and the difference was not significant.

Morris: Thank you, Dr. MUSHIN. We are at the end of our allotted two hours.

At this moment I would like to take the opportunity to digress for a moment and say, publicly, what already has been said privately; that this meeting of the World Federation is an improvement over the previous ones in its scientific aspects. I believe that this is largely due to the participation of the members in questions. You, yourselves, here this afternoon have sparked all of the discussions. I think it is also due in large part to the careful organization of the programme details by our colleague and friend, Dr. PARSLOE, at the left end side of the table.

There are signs of growth and development in our specialty. The time of taking all things on faith is behind us. We now move forward by a continual process of selection and rejection, promoted by meetings such as this. We go from here well reinforced in the need for each one of us to objectively evaluate and interpret all that we observe, being careful to avoid sweeping conclusions and spurious extrapolations. I want to give my thanks not only to the audience for their participation and close attention, but your thanks also to the Panel of experts for their entertaining and illuminating answers, some of them not easy. It appears to me that they have done very well in that most difficult of human arts – communication. It is useful to know that there is not always agreement, and that there is still room for valid differences of opinion.

Panel discussions on

C. Pediatric anaesthesia for correctable congenital anomalies

Chairman: M. DIGBY LEIGH, Los Angeles
Members: A. W. CONN, Toronto; S. IWAI, Tokyo; G. B. LEWIS, jr., Los Angeles; G. J. REES, Liverpool; R. M. SMITH, Boston.

Leigh: Dear confreres, it is a great pleasure for me to be visiting my warm-hearted South American friends. It is also an opportunity for me to renew our acquaintance with our many friends throughout the world.

In order to remind you of your own anaesthetic experiences in the neonate and to put you in the right mood, we have brought along a short movie on the neonate, completed just a month ago at the Childrens Hospital of Los Angeles. It illustrates anaesthesia in four newborn infants: 1. bilateral nephrostomy; 2. removal of a teratoma or tumour of the perineum; 3. management of intestinal obstruction, and last; 4. management of anaesthesia for esophageal atresia with fistula. Following the movie, I would like to introduce the illustrious members of our Panel. I would also request you to prepare questions and write them on a paper. Now, for the movie. "Anaesthesia in the Neonate" as done at Childrens Hospital of Los Angeles.

"In the anaesthetic management of the premature and newborn infant the following equipment is used. An infant circle filter incorporating a Revell circulator. On top of this utility cart you can see an infant blood pressure cuff and sphygmomanometer, a precordial stethoscope, a laryngoscope, endotracheal tubes in plastic wrappers, a firm suction catheter, dilute succinylcholine and atropine and an electric thermometer.

Case I: The first infant is a 6 lb. 13 oz. boy with severe bilateral hydronephrosis requiring bilateral nephrostomies. After premedication with atropine, 0.1 mg., anaesthesia is then induced with cyclopropane. Succinylcholine in a dose of 0.5 mg. per pound is then given intramuscularly and the respirations are controlled. Following relaxation of the abdominal muscles, the patient is first ventilated with oxygen and then intubated with a firm endotracheal tube. Proper placement of the tube in the trachea and not in a bronchus is indicated by symmetrical elevation of the chest and equal breath sounds. The lungs are again inflated with oxygen. In addition to adhesive strapping, the tube is also held firmly in place by the fingers. The eyes are closed and protected by clear plastic tape. Since the patient will be placed in the lateral position, a monoaural esophageal stethoscope is used to monitor the heart rate and rhythm. Maintenance of anaesthesia is with halothane and oxygen, allowing the surgeon the use of the electrocautery. The infant is placed in a circulating warm-water mattress to prevent hypothermia and the body temperature is recorded continuously from a thermister probe in the rectum. A reliable cutdown is mandatory since blood loss in excess of 40 cc. will require a blood transfusion to prevent shock in this small patient. Blood loss is replaced by the use of a syringe and a three-way stopcock. During surgery the respirations are controlled so as to provide a quiet operative field for the surgeon.

Case II: This lively neonate already has a sigmoid colostomy for treatment of an imperforate anus. Now he returns to surgery for removal of a teratoma of the perineum. Without premedication the infant is placed on a warm mattress and the blood pressure cuff and the precordial stethoscope are applied. Anaesthesia is induced with cyclopropane in a 50% concentration. The pad seen behind the shoulders extends the head and improves the airway. As an aid to intubation, succinylcholine in a dose of 4 mg. is given into the deltoid muscle. Just prior to intubation, the lungs are ventilated with oxygen and the pad is placed under the occiput. Using a straight blade, intubation is then quickly and easily performed. The endotracheal tube is a firm thin-wall # 16 French plastic tube which must be checked frequently during the operation for possible kinking or blockage by secretions. Immediately after intubation the lungs are ventilated with oxygen and the tube is secured with adhesive tape. The pad is again placed behind the shoulders and anaesthesia is continued with cyclopropane in a 20–30% concentration utilizing controlled respirations. The respirations are controlled in a rapid, shallow manner providing adequate alveolar ventilation while at the same time preventing overdistention of the alveoli and possible pneumothorax. The adequacy of ventilation is determined by the continuous infrared analysis of the end-tidal carbon dioxide concentration using a sampling catheter in the port of the endotracheal tube. Other monitors are the thermometer probe and the esophageal stethoscope.

Case III: The pad and circulating warm-water mattress are in place to receive the next infant who is a three-day-old 5 lb. 4 oz. girl with a low intestinal obstruction. The dehidration and electrolyte imbalance have been corrected by the pediatrician but the abdominal distention persists in spite of the nasogastric tube. As in all patients the heart is monitored with a blood pressure cuff and a precordial stethoscope, the latter being connected to a plastic ear mold which is worn continuously by the anaesthesiologist. The nasogastric tube is removed in order to secure a good mask fit and to prevent regurgitation around the tube. Anaesthesia is induced with cyclopropane, allowing the mouth to remain open so that the tongue will not obstruct the upper airway. As soon as the patient is unconscious and with-

out the aid of succinylcholine, the infant's trachea is intubated with a
14 French endotracheal tube. With abdominal distention and consequent
reduction in lung volume, the tidal volume is artificially increased by manual
compression of the breathing bag. With good operating conditions a large
bore catheter is inserted into the saphenous vein at the ankle. Care is taken
to make certain that the cutdown is functional and secure before the start
of surgery. Anaesthesia is maintained with cyclopropane using both
assisted and controlled respirations. The precordial stethoscope is replaced
by the more reliable esophageal stethoscope and the body temperature is
monitored and maintained near normal. During surgery abdominal relaxation is achieved by cyclopropane alone or by the use of succinylcholine
intermittently. Evisceration and handling of the intestines may cause hypotension requiring multiple small infusions of blood or concentrated albumin
to maintain the circulation. In addition, calcium gluconate is used to increase
the tone of the myocardium. Note the discrepancy in the size of the bowel
as the result of the ileal atresia.

Case IV: Over 90% of congenital esophageal atresias show these
x-ray findings. In the lateral view the lipiodol is clearly seen in the blind
upper esophageal pouch. On both films the presence of gas in the stomach
indicates a fistula between the trachea and lower esophageal segment.
Atelectasis and pneumonia are commonly present. In the premature infant
definitive repair of the esophageal atresia was delayed for fourty-eight hours
while the pneumonitis was treated. Preoperative treatment of the pulmonary
complications consists of preliminary gastrostomy under local anaesthesia,
repeated tracheobronchial aspirations, constant removal of saliva from the
upper esophageal pouch, antibiotics and placing the infant in the semi-sit-
ting position. With improvement of lung function the infant was brought to
surgery and a reliable cutdown was established under local anaesthesia.
After application of the precordial stethoscope and blood pressure cuff, the
infant is first oxygenated and then intubated awake. Succinylcholine is not
used in premature infants since these babies may have a prolonged effect of
the drug. Anaesthesia is maintained with cyclopropane using assisted and
controlled respirations. The gastrostomy tube is kept patent so that gas will
not be trapped in the stomach and intestines and consequently interfer with
both respiration and circulation. Using the extrapleural approach the fistula
is ligated followed by primary esophageal anastomosis. This approach is
associated with less postoperative pulmonary complications and reduced
mortality, especially in the premature infant; however, there is always the
possibility of a pneumothorax as a result of high airway pressure or surgical
oversight. Here, you see the infant at the end of surgery. Note that the
anaesthesiologist is holding the endotracheal tube in place. This is to prevent its accidental dislodgement which might occur even as a result of
frequent tracheobronchial aspirations performed during the operation. Also-

seen is the sampling catheter leading to the infrared carbon dioxide analyser which was used as a monitor of both respiration and circulation. The maintenance of body temperature near normal will prevent respiratory depression and possible apnea from hypothermia in the early postoperative period. In addition, it is easier to evaluate blood loss and blood replacement in a normothermic patient as compared to the cold patient with peripheral vasoconstriction, bradycardia and poor capillary refill. If the patient is hypothermic at the conclusion of surgery, nikethamide, 0.5 cc., is administered slowly intravenously. This analeptic will promote deep breathing and crying and is an excellent stir up regime for the newborn. Blood replacement is adequate in this infant as indicated by the pink colour of the skin and mucous membranes. When the infant is a small premature, the mortality rate is high. The primary causes of death are atelectasis, pneumonia or both as illustrated in this postoperative chest film. Survival depends mainly upon early and intensive postoperative care of the respiratory system. Frequent tracheobronchial aspirations may be necessary. With a precordial stethoscope in place the infant is first oxygenated and then a polyethylene catheter is passed under direct vision. An effort is made to make the patient cough. Suction is then applied and the catheter is quickly withdrawn prolonged suctioning is dangerous as hypoxia will occur. After removal of the catheter, the infant is given oxygen to breathe again."

Leigh: This film replaced the introductory remarks which are usually requested. We have a few questions ready, of course, which the Panelists prepared themselves, so I know they will be able to answer them. Now we are going to use, as an example, esophageal atresia with tracheo-esophageal fistula because it does give you many phases of anaesthesia in the neonate. Now the first question. Dr. CONN, will you be prepared to answer this one? How would you prepare for surgery a two-day-old infant with esophageal atresia who has copious saliva bubbling out of his mouth? His hands and feet are blue and there is a density in the upper right lobe of his lung.

Conn: An infant to be properly prepared, who has this complication and is two days old, requires treatment of a general nature as well as specific therapy by anaesthesiologists. In general, the first item that might be mentioned is proper positioning of the child in a semi-recumbent position. This is to prevent aspiration of secretions. The aspiration of secretions from the mouth can also be handled by inserting an esophageal tube with constant or intermittent suctioning. This infant may require anything from 12 to 18 hours of preparation. In addition, because of the findings in his chest x-ray and his apparent pneumonitis, he will certainly require antibiotics, such as penicillin (30000 units, Q. 8. H.). He also will require a cutdown, and fluid intake in an infant such as this should be low, of the order of 5 cc. per hour in a solution such as 5% glucose, 0.2% saline. There is no problem in the first day or two of replacing excess fluid loss. A newborn child can get along for two days without any fluid, if necessary, with no serious results. Because of his cyanotic extremities and pulmonary problems, the child should be placed in an Isolette, in a humidified high oxygen atmosphere. Needless to say, he must have constant good nursing care. The anaesthesiologist enters the picture more specifically, as you recently saw in the movie. He is particularly responsible for improving the lungs pre-operatively. An infant such as this would be intubated awake every half to one hour and his tracheo-bronchi suctioned. I believe that the use of suctioning through the endotracheal tube, rather than directly as you saw in the movie, is less traumatic. Before and after suctioning, the child would be oxygenated and the point of this pre-operative preparation is not only to remove secretions but to encourage the child to cough. An infant who does not cough and has this type of pathological process is likely to develop increasing pneumonitis, perhaps ending in death. The anaesthetist plays a most important role in the pre-operative preparation of these infants.

Leigh: Any comments by the rest of the Panel? Dr. LEWIS, would you have anything to add there? I think he had covered it very well. He seems to know how to handle them preoperatively.

Lewis: Many years ago I learned a very important point about the management of tracheo-esophageal fistula from Dr. PARMELEE in our hospital, who was an elderly, experienced pediatrician. He saw these patients before the days of LADD and HAIGHT, when they started doing surgery on these small babies. He said, "If you put these babies to bed and do not do any surgery on them, they will not necessarily die of their pulmonary complications, but they will die of starvation". Now, what can we do with these babies today? In a baby like this, one would think first then of nutrition and would then have a gastrostomy performed under local anaesthesia for feeding purposes. This will also help prevent regurgitation of gastric contents back up through the fistula, contaminating the lungs. Then continue with Dr. CONN's plan of taking care of the lungs, ridding them of their atelectasis and pneumonia. This can go on for days and days and when the condition has improved and the weight has increased, then think about doing the surgery.

Leigh: I think that is very good. Now, would you like to add anything, Dr. REES?

Rees: Mr. Chairman, I regret to say that I can disagree with nothing that has been said previously. But there are one or two things which I would like to add to this. The first thing is really relating to the diagnosis of the condition perhaps, and that is, I would prefer that this infant had had no radiopaque medium introduced into the esophagus, for diagnostic purposes. We would much prefer to see the diagnosis confirmed by the passage of a radiopaque catheter. The second thing which I would like to add would be that possibly an even better drainage position for the bronchial tree in this situation, is to nurse the infant in a face down or almost face-down position, that is to say, a knee-shoulder position with the head turned on to one side. This insures extraordinarily good drainage of the pharynx, and very good drainage of the bronchial tree. The third thing I would like to add, which has not been mentioned, is that if there is peripheral cyanosis, there will inevitably also be a metabolic acidosis in this child, and that part of the intravenous therapy should be directed towards the correction of this metabolic disturbance. The fourth thing which I would like to add is in relation to suction of the tracheo-bronchial tree. If the tracheo-bronchial tree needs such frequent aspiration, as has been mentioned, I would prefer to carry this aspiration out through an indwelling endotracheal tube which we would probably pass through the nose, which would enable very frequent suction to be carried out. And the fifth and final thing which I would like to mention is this question of the use of antibiotics. Now, in our institution we would give this infant antibiotics, but this would be accompanied by an extreme hazard, certainly in our center, of the development of monilia infection, which is something we fear very greatly and which we see very frequently, and although at this moment we do use antibiotics, we wonder sometimes whether the predisposition to monilia infection is not a very great disadvantage and one which might make us hesitate to do this.

Leigh: Now, JACK, I agree with you. Now, Dr. SMITH, have you anything to add?

Smith: Now it is getting down to minutia, but I think the time of operation is important, and we have two extremes here: one says do it right away; one says you can take all the time you want. Our own approach to this is to do the gastrostomy immediately. There is one reason for doing the gastrostomy right away that has not been stressed, and that is that there often is marked dilatation of the stomach that gets in the way of the respiration. This is an emergency procedure. This is the only part of the whole thing that is truly an emergency procedure, and this can be done under local anaesthesia regardless of the general condition of the baby otherwise. Now, as far as having plenty of time to do the rest of the operation, I rather disagree with that because these secretions are being formed all the time and the problem of curing the pneumonia and improving the atelectasis is a very real one. In our estimation, this should be checked as soon as the baby can possibly stand it. In the very poor-risk patients – say a premature baby of two or three pounds – we do not do the esophageal anastomosis right away, but probably the morning after admission the surgeon will go in and merely tie off the tracheo-esophageal fistula thereby controlling the secretions, and then the lung is out of its most immediate danger. After that, a small premature baby may be nursed along for many days, until he is able to withstand the whole esophageal anastomosis. This is the way we would approach the poor-risk child. The gastrostomy first, then tying off the fistula and, finally, the esophageal anastomosis.

Leigh: This is a debatable point, of course, when to do the anastomosis. I think you may find in the next few years changes in that opinion and you may find that maybe they will wait a period of time before they do the surgery. We did acid-base tests on a number of these patients with esophageal atresias and found that in most cases the acid-base balance was close to normal. Now, let us go on with the next question. We would like to know what premedication to use and we are going to ask the Panelists.

Conn: We would premedicate this child with atropine with a dosage of 0.02 mg. per kilo.

Lewis: No premedication whatsoever is necessary.

Rees: I am with Dr. Lewis, that no premedication is necessary in this case. But if you run to that, I think you would do no harm by giving atropine in a dose of about 0.1–2 mg.

Smith: I am certainly on the atropine side, partly because of the secretions, more definitely because of the drugs we are using, cyclopropane or halothane or, specially, succinylcholine. And if we are using those, specially the succinylcholine, whether we are using this intramuscularly or intravenously, I fear bradycardia, and I think the use of atropine is definitely indicated to prevent this.

Leigh: You see, we have perfect agreement in the Panel. Take your choice. You see, nothing is really settled. Our next question is what anaesthetic agent or agents would you select? Nor, Dr. Smith is very fond of local. Would you use lidocaine, Bob, for the repair?

Smith: You are misquoting me and might as well stop right here.

Leigh: I meant to.

Smith: Good. No. I would not use local.

Leigh: What would you use?

Smith: Any type of general anaesthesia with an endotracheal tube whereby I could support respiration.

Leigh: Any kind of equipment?

Smith: Any kind.

Leigh: Any agent?

Smith: Any agent probably.

Leigh: Chloroform?

Smith: No, of the popular ...

Leigh: Avertin?

Smith: All right. Cyclopropane or perhaps halothane in a strong infant, perhaps relaxants and nitrous oxide, under certain circumstances ether.

Leigh: Would you use the relaxants that we use?

Smith: I would probably use d-tubo-curarine.

Leigh: He uses d-tubo-curarine in a day-old baby.

Smith: Yes.

Leigh: JACK, do you want to support that?

Rees: Well, I do not quite know what I am supporting because there is such a wide variety of agents and techniques that have been mentioned.

Leigh: But you can choose one, can't you?

Rees: Well, I am going to say what I use, now. I think that really we must try to develop fairly clear cut ideas as to what is the method of choice, one that presents the least disadvantages, and we believe that – we may very well be wrong – but we do firmly believe that the use of potent inhalation agents in this circumstance, and indeed in all circumstances where ventilation is controlled, is perhaps undesirable. Now, the reason why I say this is, first of all, that I believe that with IPPR it is undesirable to reduce peripheral resistance, because the reduction of peripheral resistance tends to alter the distribution of blood as between the pulmonary circulation and the systemic circulation, and to alter the ventilation perfusion qualities in the lung. And the other, I think, main reason is that during IPPR the patient has no control of his ventilation rate and, in the case of drugs like halothane, therefore of the uptake of the drug which is determined by the type of ventilation minute volume which is applied. I think this adds to some extent a complication in the administration, whereas with a drug like nitrous oxide, which is not a potent drug, there is no danger of overdosage provided that an adequate provided an adequate concentration of oxygen is used. And for this reason I would use, as my anaesthetic agent, only nitrous oxide. Now, for many years, I must confess, that I would have said that the only relaxant one should use would be succinylcholine. In more recent years, as a result of pressure from below, in our department, I have been forced to revise this and I would now use d-tubo-curarine chloride as would Dr. SMITH. And at the termination of the operation, I would reverse the d-tubo-curarine chloride with neostigmine.

Leigh: You can reverse it every time completely? You noticed our patients in this film were awake and moving, and certainly did not have depressed respiration. Can you reverse it every time safely, completely? I want to hear you say this publicly.

Rees: I believe that I can reverse this every time that I want to. But on many occasions, postoperatively, especially in the type of case that you have mentioned which we are taking as an example, I would prefer not to reverse it completely at the end of the operation, because I think that child might do better if he remains postoperatively on IPPB for a number of hours or a number of days even.

Leigh: I think that IPPB for several days is certainly needed after relaxants. Dr. REES has learned to ventilate patients for very long periods of time postoperatively.

Rees: Well, of course you know quite well that Dr. LEIGH is being facetious when he says this. I believe that in all circumstances the relaxants are reversible – the non-depolarizing type of relaxant – in these cases. Provided that other factors have been corrected, that is to say biochemical, temperature of the infant and so on, have been maintained at reasonable levels. And as Dr. LEIGH is at pains to emphasize, these things are necessary in whatever combination of anaesthetic drugs is used.

Leigh: What about ALLAN CONN? What do you do in these cases?

Conn: I do not exactly disagree with Dr. REES but our method of choice would be to use a dilute solution of succinylcholine administered intravenously. Using a concentration of 1 mg. per 10 pounds of body weight per cc; one can titrate the relaxant into the child and we prefer succinylcholine because of its very brief duration and our knowledge that the child is unlikely to have a prolonged effect.

Leigh: Would you intubate all these cases of esophageal atresia?

Rees: Yes.

Smith: Unquestionably.

Leigh: All in agreement. Intubation in all of them which have an open chest. During the surgery would you aspirate the endotracheal tube? Would you aspirate frequently, Dr. REES?

Rees: I would not unless there were an indication, unless that there were evidence there were secretions to aspirate.

Leigh: Have you got anything to add, Dr. Smith?

Smith: Yes, I would go a little farther than that. Even though the stethoscope usually tells you very quickly whether or not you have secretions, you cannot have the stethoscope on all parts of the chest. And you know really, quite well, that this is probably the major problem in doing anaesthesia. I think that I would go down that trachea about at least twice during the procedure, whether or not I thought it was indicated.

Leigh: Now, we will get a little more radical. Dr. Lewis?

Lewis: I will go further than that. Even with or without atropine premedication, I would perform tracheo-bronchial suction almost every 20 or 30 minutes by the clock. Secretions will insidiously collect in your endotracheal tube and you may not be able to detect them until you have a total obstruction. Then you are in a position of having to reintubate a patient in a position that is not very favourable for intubation. He is on his side, almost face-down. Next time you take a tube out of one of these patients, look at the end of it. You will see there is a little blood, a little secretion, in spite of all the aspirations that you have done through the case.

Leigh: Dr. Conn, would you agree with anybody on the Panel so far?

Conn: I walk the fence. I do agree with suctioning if there is any evidence of secretions, but not otherwise. If, at any time, one aspirates blood, then I would agree with Dr. Lewis. There is no question that with prolonged controlled ventilation with dry gases, bleeding within the tracheo-bronchial if one aspirates a trace of blood, then I believe one is committed to automatic suctioning every 15 or 20 minutes.

Leigh: And I would advise you to take a firm catheter just a little longer than your endotracheal tube and have two or three of these because they do get blocked up. I would advise you strongly to suction every 15 minutes because you will find sometimes that there is a complete block in the end of the tube and you will not be able to remove it even with a piece of wire. So I advise you to keep out of trouble. Now, Dr. Rees, did you want to say a little more about relaxants?

Rees: Well, yes. I would like to say a little more about the properties of succinylcholine and the properties of d-tubo-curarine chloride, in this age group. Many years ago, it was described from our department, by

STEAD, that there was a greater sensitivity to d-tubo-curarine in constant weight dosage in the newly born infant than in older children and in adults. And that there was at the same time a rather greater resistance to the action of depolarizing drug like succinylcholine. And this was the reason which led us in the past to favour, as the relaxant of choice, succinylcholine for these children. But, as in other circumstances, in a myasthenic patient for instance, in adult life, in those circumstances where you tend to have a patient who, for some reason or other, is sensitive to the action of d-tubo-curarine chloride, he is at the same time prone, as in the case of the myasthenic, to develop the second phase of a competition, of a dual type of neuro-muscular block as a result of continued administration of succinylcholine. And this in fact I think is so in this age group, and that, even if one uses succinylcholine over a long period of time, it is sometimes desirable and necessary to use neostigmine to reverse the block. Now, clearly, if you are creating this situation very frequently, that is to say, using a depolarizing agent and ending up with a non-depolarizing type of block, the situation would be less complex if one had to use a non-depolarizing relaxant from the outset. And this is what led us to change practice and now to use d-tubo-curainre chloride as the relaxant of choice for operations which are to last for more than 20 minutes in this age group. But it must be remembered that these infants are more sensitive and therefore, whatever weight for weight dose is selectet of d-tubo-curarine chloride for your older patient, this must be reduced by about $1/3$ in the neonatal infant. And we titrate fractional doses 0.25 of a milligram into these infants until we produce the degree of relaxation which we consider to be desirable.

Leigh: Are you afraid of running into an atypical homozygote when you use succinylcholine? Does that bother you at all?

Rees: No, not particularly. Because this occurs in about one in four thousand of the general population. I cannot remember the figure for the incidence of esophageal atresia, but if you multiply that by the incidence of atypical homozygotes in the population, you would get an astronomical figure I would have thought.

Lewis: May I say something, Mr. CHAIRMAN?

Leigh: I cannot keep them quiet. Go ahead. It is warming up.

Lewis: Dr. REES visited us in Los Angeles and we had a wonderful two days. I learned a great deal. He taught us his technique of using d-tubo-curarine in children. We continue to try his method but I have noticed one thing about it, and that is that some of these patients, after reversal, do not have a strong cough. They cannot lift their heads. They are weak and hypotonic for some hours. This disturbs me. So, JACK, you've got to come back to Los Angeles with a better brand of neostigmine for us.

Rees: It could be, of course, that drug production in the United States of America is different from the United Kingdom, I mean, I could . . .

Leigh: He is slippery! Slippery!

Rees: . . . and I would introduce you to representatives of the drug firm. I am sure you would find it satisfactory.

Leigh: Dr. Conn wants to say something. Go ahead Allan.

Conn: In this discussion between the virtues of succinylcholine and d-tubo-curarine, a very important fact has not been mentioned. Dr. Rees, as you know, uses nitrous and oxygen with d-tubo-curare. We use nitrous oxide and oxygen but supplement N 2 O with either halothane or methoxyflurane. This reduces the total consumption of succinylcholine tremendously. The risk involved of prolonged apnea – occurring on a genetic basis once in 2,800 (in the Canadian population) – is a rare complication. The actual incidence of tracheo-esophageal atresia is close to 1 in 2000, so that an apnea is not likely to occur in more than once in, perhaps, 10 years, even in a very busy service.

Leigh: In a premature of 1,500 Gms. would you give a muscle relaxant such as d-tubo?

Rees: Yes, indeed I would. But I think that we must keep our minds clear that when we are speaking about the reversibility of relaxant drugs in these patients, and indeed in any others, and what I say of the reversibility, is applicable, I believe, only if one avoids these more potent agents. I think that other agents do have a very gross effect at the neuromuscular junction. I think this is applicable to a greater or lesser degree to most of our anaesthetic agents, and what I say about the reversibility of d-tubo-curarine chloride is only applicable if nitrous oxide is the sole agent.

Leigh: We would certainly hesitate to give a premature a muscle relaxant.

Rees: I would not.

Leigh: Would you give a relaxant, Dr. Lewis?

Lewis: Never! Never!

Leigh: Never, never give a muscle relaxant to a weak, feeble, atonic premature who is barely living, whose reflexes are poor. Now, Bob, your turn.

Smith: I think it is hard to say "never" in the face of somebody who has done it for years and gotten away with it as Dr. Rees has. Now, that is dangerous territory . . .

Conn: I think the same way about "never" . . .

Smith: . . . that I, on asked to start this discussion, I intentionally kept it rather wide, saying that almost anything could be used with care. Now, there is one thing that Dr. REES brought out that I should like to emphasize: that is the danger of giving any of the strong drugs under controlled respiration. And you are really going to get into trouble here. I think if you are giving a drug such as halothane, or cyclopropane, or ether, in controlling respiration you are going to get yourself a very deeply anaesthetized child, very easily. That is why, if you are insisting upon controlling respiration, Dr. REES makes a great deal of sense. This is also why I think it is especially dangerous to combine a relaxant with a strong agent such as cyclopropane, which is exactly in contrast with Dr. REES's ideas. So, one point I would like to leave: I would not use a strong, potent anaesthetic under controlled respiration . . . under continuous controlled respiration.

Leigh: Well, dangerous and hazardous as it is, we have used these very strong agents on these particular cases and really, BOB, we have got away with it.

Smith: Lucky.

Leigh: All right. Now, the next big problem. I know anaesthesiologists at large are not interested in monitors but I think it is most important to use monitors because the heart may stop in 30 seconds and you must know about it if you are going to have the patient survive. You should know it very, very early. Now, Dr. SMITH is going to talk about monitors because he does not believe in monitors.

Smith: Not your kind.

Leigh: Pardon?

Smith: I said "not your kind". Now, monitors are extremely important. I will not take a long time but just start this going again. I think they are extremely important. A big problem is finding out where to draw the line between too little and too much. Certainly the stethoscope is here to stay. The blood pressure apparatus is extremely important, even on these very small babies. It is the best way to tell about blood loss. The thermometer is here to stay, and that is very important, as it has been emphasized. Now, you don't see an electroencephalogram on these children, and you probably won't see the carbon dioxide analyzer on many children outside of Los Angeles. Now, to my mind, this is going a little too far in monitoring. We will have a chance to discuss this. I would like to talk about the stethoscope a little more saying that, for me, and especially on an infant, you need both ears. I insist that anybody in my hospital use a bi-aural stethoscope on these small infants, because it is hard to hear accurately. Also it is a very nice teaching instrument. You can take the stethoscope from the resident and then you can hear what he is hearing. Finally, I like to use a stethoscope that has a fairly large bell on it, because you can hear both the heart and the lungs a little better than with these tiny little stethoscopes. One other thing: usually the precordial stethoscope, even on the right side, is perhaps more satisfactory than the esophageal stethoscope. You do not know quite which side you are listening to, or where your sounds are coming from.

Lewis: I wonder if we could see slide No. 17? This is a typical anaesthetic setup as used in our hospital. Here, we see a small infant. Now, the precordial stethoscope is right there and it is attached to a piece of plastic tubing that goes to a monoaural earpiece. This is worn comfortably all day long by the anaesthesiologist. The baby has also a blood pressure cuff in place to monitor the blood pressure. Usually, we take it by the oscillometric method and notice the changes as they occur during the course of anaesthesia. The body temperature is maintained near normal by the circulating warm-water mattress placed beneath the infant. The thermometer probe is inserted into the rectum which goes back to an electronic thermometer which is nearby the anaesthesiologist. This is the heating unit supplying warm water to the mattress. Here is the BIRD mechanical ventilator and this is a BLOOMQUIST infant circle filter incorporating a REVELL circulator. This is put in the circuit so as to mix more thoroughly the anaesthetic gases and assure a fresh supply and even concentration at all times. Now, our prize, and one of our best and most reliable monitors is the infra-red carbon dioxide analyzer. This is the machine right here. The pick-up is placed in the endotracheal tube and a sample is continuously taken from the patient, passing back through into the detector head and recorded either on a scale here or on a permanent piece of paper. Now, I would like to show you, with the use of just two slides, 18 and 19, how this instrument can give you reliable information during the course of anaesthesia. Next slide No. 18. This is a baby who is on a mechanical ventilator. Notice here the uniform ventilation of the infant. Here is expiration, here is inspiration. Here is a sample of my end-expired carbon dioxide concentration which is roughly 5.5%. At this point the REVELL mechanical circulator is turned off. Look how rapidly the analyzer tells you of impending trouble. Here is one breath. Here are two breaths, three breaths, three short breaths and you know that something is wrong. Now, that is pretty fast. If you did not have this instrument on to indicate this tremendous rebreathing and the building up of carbon dioxide, you may not know respiratory acidosis was coming on for some time; maybe until it had an effect on the circulation. Then at this point, the circulator was turned on. It moves the gases around quickly at the rate of 20 or maybe 25 litres per minute, and we have a return of base line down to normal. The dead space has been removed in about two breaths. Now it is also used as a monitor of circulation. Let us see slide No. 19. Here is small baby on a mechanical ventilator. We have adequate and uniform ventilation going on all the time here. See how even and consistent this is. The surgeon was doing a patent ductus. At this point here, there was a brisk, small hemorrhage. The end-expired carbon dioxide takes a big drop, as a result of poor pulmonary capillary blood flow. With this, you have poor filling of the left ventricle and poor filling of the coronary arteries, and this is why they die so quickly even with the small amount of blood loss.

Leigh: JACK, do you want to make some comments?

Rees: I would like to make some comments on monitoring in general. My first general comment would be that, so far, the answers to this question which you received from the Panel have indicated that those who use the most potent anaesthetic agents are those who would like to have the greatest quantity of monitoring equipment surrounding them.

Leigh: It is absolutely true. We monitor from second to second.

Rees: Now, in this Panel here – I am not including myself in this group – but in this Panel here, we have the people who are regarded as the world leaders in peadiatric anaesthesia. And they are working in well equipped hospitals. The proportion however of the total number of infants born with congenital abnormalities, which they themselves can deal with in their own institutions, must be an infinitesimal proportion of the total of such infants in the world today.

Leigh: Of course . . .

Rees: Okay.

Leigh: . . . of course, I am deeply impressed with the number of people employed in the recovery rooms of Dr. REES and Dr. CONN; fantastic number, 15 or 20. Two people for each patient. Isn't it so?

Rees: Yes.

Leigh: And what are the chances of these patients breathing on their own?

Rees: Continuing my dissertation, I would say that we have a responsibility as leaders – I do not regard myself as a leader – but the other Panelists have a responsibility to reduce this paediatric anaesthesia to its simplest terms. And to reduce its complexity to a way in which satisfactory methods can be applied in all corners of the world. And I believe that if the anaesthetic technique is kept simple and a minimum number of agents are used, then you can reduce the number of contingencies which will arise during the course of that anaesthesia, and therefore reduce the amount of monitoring and pieces of monitoring equipment which are necessary. I do agree with Dr. SMITH – I think you said temperature was important – I think this is eminently important. But you can measure temperature, preferably by an electronic thermometer, but you can measure temperature by a much simpler method with a mercury thermometer. And I think temperature must be monitored. I think peripheral circulation must be monitored, visually or, if you are lucky enough, by some sort of transducer which will measure peripheral pulsation. And I think that blood loss must be monitored very carefully. And I think that, provided a simple anaesthetic technique is used, and provided that these parameters are carefully measured, and if deviations in their values occur, they are corrected. I think that is enough to carry on. Now, our aim should be to develop anaesthetic techniques which need the minimum of monitoring, not to introduce anaesthetic techniques which demand such complex equipment to avoid the pitfalls and hazards of those complex methods.

Leigh: Did you see what we feel? In the operating room we might use more potent anaesthetic agents, but in the recovery room our patients would survive and breathe spontaneously much sooner than Dr. REES's. He forgets about the relaxant. We believe that the relaxant and nitrous oxide is no different than using stronger agents and having more rapid recovery. So you see, we are together really because he is using just as potent agents as we are.

Rees: Now, what we were discussing really was monitoring, at that moment.

Conn: Two points occurred to me during the discussion of the past two or three minutes. One: I hope none of the members of the audience would insert an esophageal stethoscope during the repair of the TE-fistula. It is quite apparante what the problems technically would be, but there is need for a stethoscope on the outside of the chest. Secondly, in the argument of blood pressure cuffs versus intra-arterial canulas, etc., I would like to stress the importance of observing the oscillation of the needle using an air manometer. An oscillometer is extremely valuable because, when the oscillations diminish, one appreciates that the stroke volume and the degree of vascular resistance has changed and that the child presumably needs more blood. I would suggest that you do not use mercury blood pressure manometers because they are not as sensitive, and that air manometers, although not as absolutely accurate, are much more practical for measuring the patients blood pressure.

Leigh: Now, one more point. You were going to say something about blood replacement, Bob?

Smith: Dr. CONN mentioned the importance of having an intravenous cutdown at the start. I am sure this is most important. We are getting into the use of plastic needles in many children now, but this does not include the small infant I am sure. A good cutdown is especially important. How much blood do you give these patients? This is a big problem. Usually there is not rapid or brisk hemorrhage during a tracheoesophageal fistula. I think you can probably stay within the old rule of 10 cc. per pound and this will usually carry you through. In addition to that however, you should go on some signs: you should have your sponges where they can be seen, and so you can estimate the blood on the sponges as they are removed. You should watch the volume of the pulse: that will tell you if there is blood loss, and the volume of the pulse will diminish. I have always thought that the volume of the heart sound was a very important thing: as a marked blood loss occurs, the heart sound will be lost to your ears, and as the blood is replaced, this will come back. I think now, however, that the use of the blood pressure cuff in a small infant is our best guide. The colour of the skin, even the colour of the lips, and especially the colour of the fingers is most misleading. I have seen children bleed to death, and still have pink fingertips. On the other hand, I think the colour of the conjunctivae is an excellent sign, except that you do not like, in these small infants, to keep prying their eyes open. And, in the small infant, I do not use this sign.

Leigh: Would you like to say a word about the value of the venous pressure or palpitation of the veins at the base of the neck to make sure that there is adequate blood to fill the heart or if there is not too much blood overdistending the heart? Would you like to say a word about that?

Smith: I agree. You certainly can get into trouble by giving too much blood, and that you should watch for venous distention. Of course these children are all covered by drapes, and that is difficult to find. But in the scalp, or the head, these may protrude individually, or you may get flushing. I think another sign is a dull slowing heart beat, that you can sometimes hear audibly or see.

Leigh: Now, Dr. IWAI, remember, has only been back in Japan three years doing pediatric anaesthesia.

Iwai: I would like to show a picture of a few of children who had tracheoesophageal fistula at birth. These patients had operation during 1962. May I see number 43 slide? This is a little dark. We have done eight cases of congenital esophageal atresia with fistula in 1962. This picture was taken last year. We are checking all survived cases every year for the development of them. This one, every time I see her I feel so happy because she is the smallest one we had. She was 1500 gm. at the operation. The surgeon did one-stage repair of the esophagus. We had enough troubles with her. May I see number 41 slide? This was taken the second day of post-operation. You can see the atelectasis of the right lung. We usually do tracheo-bronchial toilet for the treatment of atelectasis. That is, we intubate the baby first, and put 0.5 to 1.0 ml of normal saline into, and suck them out and give gentle inflation. We did this procedure several times for her. We are using an infant feeding tube – very soft one – for suction, because hard suction tube may make a hole in the lung. Unfortunately, I made a hole in the lung of this baby. Next slide number 42 please. You can see the pneumothorax. Four hours after I did tracheo-bronchial toilet, nurse told me, she does not breathe well and respiratory rate increasing. So I went down to the hospital and saw the baby. Respiratory rate was over 70 but not cyanotic. I noticed that right side of her chest did not move during respiratory cycle. I heard respiratory sound of right side, I think it might be an echo from other side. Next morning, the surgeon did closed thoracotomy and tremendous effort were paid over a month. And fortunately we made it.

Leigh: That's good. Very good, Dr. Iwai from Tokyo. Now, you see, they are making a very good point here. Very seldom do you see a spontaneous pneumothorax in a premature, because they are not strong enough to make a hole in their lungs. Isn't that true, Bob? Dr. Hingson who has had vast experience in this field corroborates this. He says very seldom do you see a pneumothorax in a premature because they are not strong enough to blow a hole. Now, we have to congratulate you, Dr. Iwai, on this excellent series. Subglottic edema in the newborn does not occur from endotracheal intubation, does it? Bob, did you ever see it?

Smith: Very rarely.

Leigh: Did you ever see it? Just about never in the newborn. Just like ventricular fibrillation; it seldom occurs in the newborn. Now, do you want to talk more about pulmonary complications? Let Dr. Lewis say one word about the mortality and what to expect in these cases. Now, Dr. Lewis is going to point out to you that it is not necessarily how you do the anaesthesia. No, that is not nearly as important as another feature.

Lewis: In a little study of survival rates in the operation for esophageal atresia, 110 cases were reviewed. These cases show a definite relationship between body weight and survival rate. In infants less than 1.5 kg, we have no survivals. Up to 1.5 and 2 kg you start having survivals at the rate of about 35%. Then up to 2 and 2.5 kg, it is about 45%. From 2.5 to 3 kg, it is about 65%. See, as the weight goes up, more babies live and by the time you have a full term, 3 kg and otherwise healthy newborn, the survival rate is 95%.

Leigh: So you see, all this discussion has been for nothing. It does not matter what you use if you have a full-term baby with no anomalies; 95% should survive. Now, that covers that and we are going to change the topic. As an example of the management of anaesthesia in the newborn, we have used the tracheo-esophageal fistula because there are so many complications and, as you noticed, most are pulmonary and have to be attended to. Now, we are going to move on to the diaphragmatic hernia. ALLAN, have you some results from your hospital?

Conn: May we have slide number 8, please? In preparation for this program, we reviewed our series and this is last year's mortality rate. This slide illustrates merely one point: the mortality rate in congenital diaphragmatic hernia at our hospital is 30%.

Leigh: We have a high mortality rate in diaphragmatic hernia and Dr. LEWIS is going to point out why these patients die.

Lewis: May I have slide number 13, please. I must congratulate Dr. CONN on his good mortality rate. Ours is much higher than that, approaching 50%. Now, I would like to point out why this rate is so high. This is an autopsy specimen of one of our diaphragmatic hernias. Let me point out to you the lung. Here is the left lung, here is the right. Now, as the intestines come up into the chest, the viscera compress that lung. It becomes totally atelectatic, unaerated and hypoplastic. The lung on the other side has to carry the load but it has trouble, too, as there are areas of atelectasis and emphysema on this side. Now, when you look at these lungs in a more careful manner, you will find another very interesting point. Slide number 14, please. In a study of these lungs, we see that the weight of a normal lung combines to a total of 50 gms., in a normal newborn. Now, the lungs in a patient with diaphragmatic hernia are small. They are hypoplastic and they weigh but only 17 gms. as compared to the normal of 50 gms. Now, out of that lung that weighs 17 gms., the left one is unaerated, nonfunctional, and so life is maintained by this little 13 gms. lung. This is not enough functioning lung tissue for these patients to survive and this is why they die. Now, let us look at the next slide a minute. No. 15, please. Now, we try to find out just how we can help these patients who have a severe lung disease. We did some ASTRUP techniques on these patients and found out that with their severe lung problem, they not only had hypoxia and cyanosis but that they had a marked respiratory acidosis and a metabolic acidosis as indicated by the pH of 7.022 at the beginning of the anaesthesia. Note here the high PCO_2 at the start of anaesthesia and the negative value for the base excess. This indicates a mixed and severe respiratory acidosis and metabolic acidosis. Now, 24 hours later, after surgery, there is an improvement of the patient with an elevation of the pH to 7.3. The PCO_2 had fallen to a lower level and the base excess was at a normal value. Now, there is a similarity between the patient with diaphragmatic hernia and hyaline membrane. They both have this type of acid-base setup. They both have decreased functioning lung tissue and they both have a self-limiting disease which, if you get them over 4 or 5 days, will survive. With this thought in mind, we planned an approach of therapy using HUTCHINSON's idea of giving these babies more frequent ASTRUP titrations and then infuse sodium bicarbonate to correct the severe acidosis.

Leigh: We find that the determination of the acid-base status is important. When the pH gets below 7, watch out! There will be more potassium in the blood and the heart will come to a standstill.

Rees: I would like to say a little word to emphasize what Dr. LEWIS has been saying about the conditions of the lung's condition in diaphragmatic hernia. He said that the reason why the lung in this condition was small was because the abdominal contents prevented its development. Well, now, I am not at all sure that this is absolutely true because in a very small proportion of these diaphragmatic hernias you find an abnormal lung on the contra-lateral side as well, which rather suggests that the lung pathology is probably a primary phenomenon in its own right, and it could even be that the diaphragmatic hernia is a feature which is secondary to the lung abnormality.

Leigh: That is a very good point, Jack, because you see, it seems to support the figures of BUTLER and SNYDER that the lung is not fully developed. Now, JACK, do you mind showing us that delightful film on how you manage the newborn postoperatively. He has a delightful film here and I would like him to show it to you. I think you will like it.

Rees: Now, this film actually has already been shown by my colleague, Dr. STEAD, at this Congress, but there were not so very many people there. And it is relevant, and Dr. STEAD has allowed me to put this on this morning here. It shows the postoperative respiratory management as we now carry it out on neonatal infants.

Leigh: You know, JACK, don't apologize for showing a film fifty times because the first time they see it, what they only see is the colour. Before you can follow the technique of Dr. REES accurately, you will have to look at this film ten to twenty times. Do not say "I have seen that film". You have not seen it because in a film new things occur every time you see it. All right, show the film now. It is a new idea, too. That is why I want you to know about it. I think it was developed by Dr. DURHAM SMITH of Adelaide, wasn't it?

Rees: Yes, yes. The idea of this film, which has no sound track, is to show that it is quite possible to carry out prolonged IPPB on small infants. This infant is not a postoperative case; I might say it is an infant who had broncho-pneumonia. Now, it is not necessary to do tracheostomies in order to carry out prolonged IPPB. This child has a soft plastic portex, naso-tracheal tube, and it has been shown by ALLAN that you can leave such tubes in for certainly as long as two months without producing any significant laryngeal damage. We have devised a special tube for this purpose, with the cross-piece which you saw, which enables the inspiratory and the ex-piratory limbs of the respirator to be connected to this tube – there will be detailed shots of these shortly – and enables the IPPB to be carried out with this monster which we use sometimes. The important thing, if one is to leave a tube in for a long time, is to insure that the humidification of the gases is 100% at body temperature, at the patient's mouth. This involves a heated humidifier, which we thermostat to about 55° centrigrade. And the tubing between there and the patient is of a plastic material, so there is very little heat loss, and at the patient's mouth, the endotracheal tube, the tem-perature is about 37°. The tube is designed in such a way that the connect-ions to the ventilator can be permanently attached to the endotracheal tube – the tube has a cross-piece – and when the inspiratory limb is attached to one side of the cross, the expiratory limb to the other, the prolongation of the tube down the nose and down the trachea is plugged off normally, but for a tracheo-bronchial toilet can be readily removed. This sort of setup with the tubings rigidly fixed to the child's head greatly facilitates nursing and mobility of the child – and mobility of the child is an essential part of management, of course, when a child is on prolonged IPPB. This child was maintained on the ventilator by the use of narcotics – not by the use of relaxants – but they are sometimes used by us. And you see this type of endotracheal tube makes aspiration of the bronchial tree very simple and much more readily performed aseptically, I think, than tracheo-bronchial toilet through a tracheostomy, which is the alternative to this if you are faced with circumstances where prolonged IPPB is necessary. And you see that, for suction, it is simply a question of removing the plug by some sort of non-touch technique using disposable forceps, passing the suction catheter way down the endotracheal tube. Well, now, some of these cases of diaphragmatic hernia, with inadequate pulmonary tissue for the maintenance of life, do in fact need this sort of management postoperatively.

And indeed do many other cases following surgery in early life, some esophageal atresias with a lot of bronchial aspirations preoperatively, they will also be treated in this way. This is the tube, demonstrated: you see that the cross-piece enables the inspiration limb and the expiratory limb to be attached to the patient with no dead space at all virtually, because what corresponds to the Y piece of the ventilator is integrated into the endotracheal tube.

Leigh: Delightful film and beautifully narrated. Now, JACK, would you use this on a patient with hyaline membrane disease or what they now call respiratory distress syndrome?

Rees: Some of our boys have had one or two cases treated like this. Only, hyaline membrane disease is a tremendous problem because you have this unstable condition of the lung as a result of the defective surface active substance, and I am not quite sure that . . . I think the hyaline membrane disease is still a problem which we have got to face and solve. I think that IPPB is the best we have to offer at this moment, but I do not think that it is the ultimate by any means.

Leigh: As Dr. REES points out, it gets away from a tracheostomy which you know is a very serious thing in a newborn, particularly because the glottis does not grow unless it is used. Use and disuse are important in growth or in failure of growth of the glottis.

Conn: I want to show a slide to prove that this technique is not used solely in Australia or in Britain. Can we have slide No. 4? Slide No. 4 is a picture of a child with respiratory distress, who is in the Isolette, and being "serviced", if you like, by a BIRD respirator in "Q" circle. Can we now have slide No. 5, which is a close-up of the same infant. As you can see, he is being monitored as much as possible. For the postoperative cases that do not require Isolette, I will show you slide No. 6, please. This is a good respirator which is adapted to an infant's crib by having its own sling. Again the child is on "Q" circle system which has a dead space of, supposedly, 0.6 cc. and, in slide 7, you see that same infant up close. It is quite easy to suction through that little cap at the top. These children require usually no drug therapy to maintain controlled respirations on the ventilator. They are fully awake and they can swallow. This technique may be used up to ages 10 and 12 years, for acute postoperative problems, The children are fully conscious with respirations being assisted or controlled by nasal intubation and artificial respiration. Lights, please.

Leigh: Now, another very interesting operation is an omphalocele and I think, BOB, you wanted to say something about that.

Smith: With omphalocele the difficulty that we have is almost entirely because of what the surgeon does, as you know. A child with a large omphalocele has this great mass out in front of his abdomen. The surgeon pushes it back in and forces the diaphragm way up, and the baby cannot breathe. This is our entire problem. And we have various methods of overcoming this. We usually intubate the patient. Some of us believe in using a relaxant so that we can give the surgeon maximum relaxation. Some believe in keeping the child breathing all the time. Now, whether you do this or not, the most important problem is maintaining respiration after the operation. Now, what can the surgeon do to help you out? There are other methods other than stitching the abdomen up. May I have slide No. 35, please. This shows one technique which has been used in a number of hospitals in North America, and that is shown on this child on the left. If you simply paint a large omphalocele with mercurochrome – I do not know whether it is the mercury or just the drying solution of the alcohol – but a large omphalocele will gradually dry up and contract and heal over. And this overcomes the necessity of this immediate difficulty in operation. This has been used in a number of different clinics with success, even on some of the largest omphaloceles. And I think it is worthy of trial in a large scale. May I have the next slide, please? Now this is the other problem which, again, is surgical but does confront us. Sometimes the surgeon has difficulty in closing the muscle wall, and only closes the skin over the lesion and then discharges the child having him come back later. This is a moderately large one – it may be even larger. If you delay the closure of this omphalocele in this method, it may become literally impossible to reduce this and repair the lesion, because the liver, as well as other viscera, will continue to bulge outward and the rectus muscles will form almost a board-like iron band across the posterior part of the abdomen. And when you go to reduce this and put the liver back underneath the rectus muscles, the rectus muscles will not give and you compress the inferior vena cava as well as the aorta and the patient may die on the table. Some of these patients just cannot be repaired if they are left in this way. So you are faced with the method of reducing these patients at the time of operation. Now, in our hospital, one of the best improvements in the last few years has been a method of closure of these large omphaloceles in the newborn – may I have the next slide, please – the following one – by a plastic envelope. Here is a picture of a large omphalocele and, around the omphalocele, which cannot be closed, is a teflon envelope. This encircles the omphalocele at the time of operation, and this is drawn moderately snug, but there is very little pressure. This child will not have difficulty in the postoperative period. About four days later, this child will come back for operation, and this envelope will be tightened and probably half of it can be removed and thrown away, and the child will be sent back to the ward. Then, another three days later, perhaps the final stage – it may take two or three different operations. But at each one of these operations there will be no difficulty, postoperatively, for the patient to breathe. Now, this, to me, has been one of the major improvements in solving a very nasty problem for the anaesthetist. And if you can have your surgeon learn this staged closure of an omphalocele, I think this will overcome, as I say, one of our most difficult problems in postoperative management. Thank you.

Leigh: As you heard Dr. Smith say, occasionally the heart will stop even in this newborn. I am sure that we know it is a rare affair for the newborn to have cardiac arrest on the table.

Smith: In operations for omphalocele you are looking for signs of circulatory embarrassment. The first thing you will get, when the surgeon starts to push this into the abdomen, obviously will be a decrease in peripheral return, but you cannot see that in a patient under drapes. So you have a stethoscope there and you may get an initial slowing of the heart. If it goes that far, naturally you immediately tell the surgeon to release his closure and at once the baby's heart should pick up, if you carry it this far.

Leigh: Suppose it stops?

Smith: Digby wants me to talk about cardiac ressuscitation. In an infant on the table, the first thing you do, of course, is continue to ventilate. But don't over-ventilate. We may get excited and ventilate too hard, and that is almost worse than not at all, because you prevent returning venous circulation, which is bad anyway. So, ventilate slowly, maybe 12 times a minute, even in a small child. But fully. And then relax and let the heart return. If, in this first second or two, you notice this, of course you compress the heart. It is very simply done providing you are in an operation where the surgeon has the chest open, naturally he compresses that heart. If, in a case like this he does not, you can simply reach under the drapes yourself. Here is the child: put your finger, or thumb, on top of the chest, your hand underneath – very simple to compress the heart in this direction, in this method. It is better, I think, than going down like this, which drives the child into the bed or table. Put your hand underneath and compress it. Again, the rate would be probably 36, 40 times a minute. This you can overdo. Do it calmly if you can, and don't overdo it, don't get exited.

Leigh: Is that all you are going to do? How do you know there is any blood in that heart?

Smith: I am not going to give him coramine, I tell you that . . .

Leigh: In my experience there is often no blood in the heart so you've got to put some blood in that heart. At times the veins are empty; the blood is in the extremities and the viscera.

Lewis: Dr. SMITH mentioned poor venous return and this deserves some treatment. You must place these patients head down and elevate the legs. This will increase venous return. One can also administer blood through a cutdown.

Leigh: You should lift up the legs and maybe put a little pressure on the abdomen so as to fill the heart with blood, because you can't pump an empty heart. Would you give any drugs, now?

Smith: Calcium gluconate or chloride, about 1 cc. would be 100 mg. in a small infant, and I also like epinephrine. And these children tolerate relatively large doses of epinephrine, I think primarily because they are anoxic and acidotic. A few years ago we were very scared about giving such large doses of 1:1000 epinephrine, but, I am sure, it is better to give it quickly and give it fairly concentrated, than wait a long time and worry about mixing it up. I think probably about a quarter, a fifth of one cc. of 1:1000 epinephrine in a child whom you are having a hard time to start the heart is indicated, and useful and not dangerous.

Leigh: We are very sorry our time is up and we have only touched on the subject. We are just merely giving you a smattering so that you would be interested in the subject. The Panelists and I wish to thank you for being such an enthusiastic and attentive audience. Good bye, good health and happiness to my wonderful friends of Brazil and all other countries.

D. The mechanism of action of local anaesthetics

Chairman: P. R. BROMAGE, Montreal
Members: E. K. ERIKSSON, Upplands-Väsvy; I. C. GEDDES, Liverpool;
A. P. TRUANT, Worcester; J. E. USUBIAGA, Buenos Aires; L. S. WOLFE,
Montreal.

Section I.

Basic actions of local anaesthetics on excitable tissues

Chairman: Our knowledge of the fundamental actions of local anaesthetics has increased greatly during the past twenty years, but much of the recent data is scattered through the literature of several disciplines, and the time has come to bring these different streams of information together. The function of our panel is to act as a focal point for some of this scattered information, and we will try to bridge the gap between recent advances in basic science and their application in the clinical field.

The members of the panel have been chosen for their different roles in this synthesis. Dr. LEON WOLFE who is Chief of Neurochemistry at the Montreal Neurological Institute, will introduce us to the ground floor of the problem and see to it that our feet are planted on as firm biophysical ground as possible in the present state of knowledge.

Dr. ALDO TRUANT, Director of Astra Research Laboratories at Worcester, Massachusetts, is well known for his work on local anaesthetics and isolated nerve preparations, and he will deal mainly with structure-function relationships.

The rest of us are clinicians. Dr. EJNAR ERIKSSON is primarily a surgeon with special interests in local anaesthesia, neuroanaesthesia and the physiology of Arctic survival. Dr. ERIKSSON has made some outstanding contributions to the clinical aspects of local anaesthesia, and we will ask him to deal with questions of ionic environment and the disposition and excretion of local anaesthetics.

Dr. IAN GEDDES from the University of Liverpool has made very careful studies of the breakdown and excretion of local anaesthetics within the body, using radioactive tracer techniques, and he will also deal with questions of excretion and toxicity.

Dr. Jose Usubiaga from Buenos Aires has made a number of valuable contributions to the South American literature on the transfer of local anaesthetics across the dura mater, as well as the enzymatic relationships of local anaesthetics and the muscle relaxants. Dr. Usubiaga will deal with some of the effects of local anaesthetics on the central nervous system and on the skeletal musculature.

My own part is to see that the title of this panel is interpreted in terms of a dynamic rather than a static relationship between local anaesthetic drugs and the tissues, because the effects of these drugs are determined to a large degree by the conditions of the tissues into which they are introduced. These conditions may alter within a wide range, and while some of the deviations from the normal (such as those associated with arteriosclerosis or pregnancy) may be beyond our control, others are within our power and are amenable to acute change. Thus, one of the important tasks of this panel will be to emphasize the elements of control that do exist, and the modifications of local anaesthetic action that can be achieved by manipulating the internal environment.

The panel will be conducted on a question-and-answer basis, and for the benefit of the audience two projectors and two screens will be used. One will project the participants' illustrations in the usual way, and on the other one we will project the question that is being answered by the panel at any particular time.

We will begin by asking Dr. Wolfe to discuss the molecular basis for conduction blockade.

Wolfe (1) *Site of action*

Research over a number of years has clearly shown that the site of action of local anaesthetics and general anaesthetics is at the surface membrane of cells of excitable tissues, more particularly at the nodes of Ranvier and postsynaptic membranes.

In vitro studies have shown that local anaesthetics can inhibit glycolytic metabolism [1, 2]. In Table 1 the lowest concentrations of several local anaesthetics which inhibit glycolysis and sodium and potassium ion trans-

Table 1. *Concentration of local anaesthetics in moles/litre which inhibit cation transport and metabolism compared to anaesthetic potency.*

	Procaine	Lidocaine	Cocaine	Tetracaine	Dibucaine
Inhibition of cation transport	1.1×10^{-2}	6.1×10^{-3}	5.3×10^{-3}	1.2×10^{-3}	7.9×10^{-5}
Inhibition of metabolism	1.8×10^{-2}	4.3×10^{-3}	5.0×10^{-4}	9.7×10^{-4}	1.2×10^{-5}
Anaesthesia	7.6×10^{-3}	2.3×10^{-3}	1.3×10^{-3}	6.0×10^{-4}	4.2×10^{-4}

port [3, 4] are compared with anaesthetic concentrations. Only in the case of cocaine and dibucaine is the concentration required for anaesthesia greater than the minimal concentrations inhibiting metabolism. In contrast local anaesthetics have little effect on the oxygen uptake of metabolizing brain tissue slices [5]. Many depressant drugs interfere with cell oxidations but functional anaesthesia is not always attended by depressed respiration. A metabolic system can be inhibited by a non-specific physicochemical interaction of the foreign molecules with the mitochondrial membrane as well as by a specific inhibition of enzymes in a biochemical reaction. The inhibition of overall respiration or of individual enzymes is not peculiar to anaesthetic agents; convulsants are also inhibitors. While it is certainly true that inhibition of oxidation often accompanies anaesthesia it does not seem to be the cause of it. LARRABEE [6] has found that with the isolated perfused ganglion preparation a five times greater concentration of local anaesthetic was required to depress resting metabolism than was required for synaptic block. Local anaesthetics do interfere with the normal sodium fluxes occurring during the generation of a nerve impulse. However, inhibition of active sodium efflux (i.e. the sodium pump) is probably not responsible for clinical anaesthesia [7]. The maintenance of the resting membrane potential of nerves does depend on oxidative metabolism which restores and maintains the ionic distributions across the excitable membrane. Local anaesthetics do not affect the membrane potential [8]. In fact they reduce the depolarization that is induced by metabolic inhibition.

Thus we must look elsewhere for understanding of the cellular site and mechanism of action of local anaesthetics. It is quite apparent that local anaesthetics in some way alter the surface membrane characteristics which are related to the generation and maintenance of nerve impulses. This brings us into the complex field of membrane structure and properties. Unfortunately our knowledge of the chemical composition and stereochemistry of any cell membrane is fragmentary. The next great and looming problem of molecular biology is the elucidation of structure and function of cell membranes. At present it is impossible even to attempt a molecular description of the surface of any cell, far less of the nodes of RANVIER or the pre- and postsynaptic membranes. Yet it is in this area that the descriptions of anaesthetic action in molecular terms will almost certainly be made. A few simple comments on membrane structure and properties are necessary before considering the effects of local anaesthetics on ion fluxes across the nerve membrane.

The cellular membrane is essentially a hydrated lipid-protein-carbohydrate complex. It is a dynamic and highly labile structure which is capable of reversible configurational transformations. These transformations result in changes in geometry, structure and phase of the lipid-protein micelles [*see* 9]. Table 2 summarizes in simple chemical terms the main constituents

of membranes and the general properties of the functional groups which
can interact with other membrane constituents or with biological or foreign
molecules.

Table 2. *Constituents of cell membranes.*

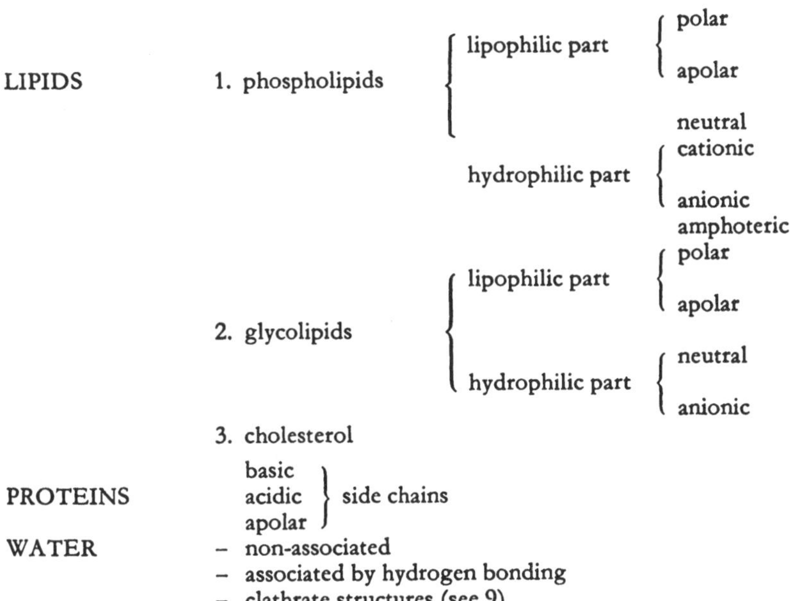

It is a remarkable fact that despite many attempts, the existence of true
covalent or chemical bonds other than hydrogen bonding between lipids
and proteins in biological membranes has not been demonstrated. It appears that membrane lipid-protein associations are held together entirely by
physicochemical forces. Table 3 lists the main types of these forces involved
in maintenance of membrane structure. Electrostatic forces are the important
forces in bringing lipids and proteins together and VAN DER WAALS forces
in holding the lipids together through their hydrocarbon side chains.
Hydrogen bonds are important stabilizing forces in protein orientations.
Water of course can compete in hydrogen bonding. Hydrophobic bonds
are very important in stabilizing complexes between the apolar groups of
lipids and protein in the membrane structure and also with the apolar groups
of foreign molecules like local anaesthetics reacting on the hydrated membrane surface.

It is generally agreed today that the cell membrane can be represented
in a rough model as a bimolecular lipid leaflet between layers of protein.
This is the classical DAVSON-DANIELLI model [10]. This structure may be
penetrated by pores or channels which are hydrophilic and charged. The

Table 3. *Physicochemical cohesion forces in membranes.*

1. Electrostatic	ion-ion interactions e.g. anionic lipid with cationic side chain group of protein. The energy varies as $1/D$ (distance)
2. Polarization	ion-induced dipole, permanent dipole-induced dipole interactions e.g. interactions between cholesterol hydroxyl group and apolar protein side chains (serine). The energy varies as $1/D^4$
3. London-Van der Waals Dispersion	transient dipole – induced dipole interactions due to the average of molecular interactions involving instantaneous changes in dispersion, induction and orientation. These quantum mechanical forces are always attractive. e.g. interactions between apolar hydrocarbon side chains of phospholipid fatty acids. The attraction energy for dispersion and induction effects varies as $1/D^6$ whereas that residing in orientation as $1/D^3$
4. Hydrophobic bonding	Hydrocarbon chains in an aqueous environment lead to the ordering of water molecules around the chains, restricting their motion. So-called iceberg or clathrate structures.
5. Hydrogen bonding	weak chemical bonds resulting from the attraction of two electronegative groups for a proton (H^+). The energy increases with the electronegativity of the two bonded molecules e.g. interactions between two carboxyl groups.

1 and 2 are sometimes referred to as polar bonds and 3 and 4 as non-polar bonds.

diameter of these channels has been estimated to be about 2 Å in the resting state increasing to 3–4 Å in the activated state. The hydrated sodium cation has a diameter of 3.4 Å. The pores would occupy only about 1/10,000 th of the total membrane surface area. The strongest evidence for the DAVSON-DANIELLI model has come from electron microscopic studies [11]. The surface membrane appears as a triple layered structure about 100 Å thick. Further, STOECKENIUS has demonstrated that lipoprotein films on air-water interfaces have a similar appearance in the electron microscope [12]. Caution is needed, however, in taking the electron microscopic evidence as the last word in membrane structure. It leaves unexplained many properties of the cell membrane particularly the active surfaces of neurones. Most physical measurements so far have been made across the membrane. No radial periodicities suggesting pores are seen, but they are probably too small for resolution and furthermore may not be there all the time. What is urgently needed is study in the plane of the membranes and this is particularly pertinent to anaesthetic action. FERNANDEZ-MORAN [13, 14] has started work in this area using low-temperature electron microscopy. In the mitochondrial membrane regular spherical or polyhedral repeating units are seen embedded in a hydrated lipoprotein framework. It is to be hoped that soon the surface appearance of the nodal membrane and the subsynaptic membrane will be visualized. Recent high resolution electron-microscopic studies indicate that the synapse may have a complex web-like structure.

The cell membrane may be visualized as an ever-changing mosaic between limits defined by the nature of their constituents and their inter and intra-molecular interactions which can be activated or inhibited by biological or foreign small molecules. Some of the characteristics of cell membranes, particularly those of the nerve cell are listed in Table 4.

Table 4. *Characteristics of the cell membrane.*

1. Hydrated lipid-protein	carbohydrate complex.
2. Multiphasic	the lipid bilayer can be interdigitated by protein or carbohydrate producing channels with fixed ionic sites.
3. Polyionic	
4. Mosaic	probably dependant by a genetically determined protein pattern.
5. Dynamic	transitions between semi-fluid and semi-rigid substructures. Has statistical sieve-like properties, the activated pores for Na^+ must be at least 3.4 Å and for K^+ 2.2 Å in diameter.
6. Spontaneously coalesce	probably like the coalescence phenomenon of mixed phospholipid coacervates.
7. Electrically excitable	the assumption of two stable states when a fixed potential is applied to the membrane. Nerve cells are both excitable and regenerative.

After this brief summary of membrane properties let us examine the more specific effects of local anaesthetics on nervous tissue. As has been mentioned already local anaesthetics do not alter the membrane potential, capacitance or resistance [8, 15, 18]. In some studies a slight hyperpolarization has been found. Local anaesthetics stabilize cell membranes in the same way as high external calcium concentrations, and they reversibly block the activated increase in membrane sodium conductance whether of electrical or neurohumoral origin. The stabilization theory of SHANES is really a modification of LILLIE's earlier permeability theory of anaesthetic action and regards stabilizer molecules as restricting permeability by a surface obstruction effect. Substances increasing permeability to sodium and potassium are labilizers and depolarize the membrane e.g. low calcium, potassium, veratrine, chloroform, ether. It is probably more correct to consider stabilizer and labilizer drugs as molecules which alter membrane intermolecular forces to produce a tightening or loosening of membrane structure [16]. Thus local anaesthetics through surface combination may inhibit the increase in sodium permeability normally produced by excitation by a combination with the surface membrane which alters the balance of physiochemical forces of the membrane constituents. Table 5 summarizes some of the most important effects of local anaesthetics on physiological processes in nerve. With low concentrations of local anaesthetics a partial nerve block can be produced. In these circumstances low frequency impulses are transmitted across the block whereas high frequency impulses are not. This is known as Wedensky inhibition and is due to an increase in the length of the refractory period. The studies of Condouris [17] illustrate clearly the competition between local anaesthetics and external sodium. There is a much greater susceptibility to cocaine block if surrounding fluids are low in sodium. In many ways the effects of low external sodium on nerve are similar to local anaesthetic action.

Table 5. *Effects of local anaesthetics on excitable tissues.*

1. Produce reversible non-depolarizing block.
2. Depress the rate of rise and amplitude of the action potential.
3. Lower the conduction velocity and cause decremental conduction.
4. Impede transmission of repetitive discharges.
5. Anodal polarization relieves the block.
6. Reduce Na^+ entry.
7. Reduce K^+ outflux.
8. Reduce the depolarization induced by metabolic inhibition.
9. Competitively antagonized by Na^+.
10. Antagonized by increase in external calcium.

In brief – Reversibly block the activated increase in membrane Na^+ conductance caused by excitation.

Besides effects on peripheral nerves local anaesthetics in appropriate concentrations cause marked depression of neuronal activity in the central nervous system. This effect appears due to an interference in the transmitter-sensitive component of the subsynaptic membrane. Depression of the excitatory postsynaptic potentials by anaesthetic agents is probably due to non-specific membrane stabilization to the depolarizing effects of acetylcholine [19].

Nothing is known of the real nature of the receptor molecules for local anaesthetics on nerve or the subsynaptic membrane. Ehrenpreis [20] has isolated a 'receptor-protein' from the electroplaques of electric eels which precipitates in the presence of local anaesthetics. These studies may well have pertinence to the important issue of the type of membrane component reacting with local anaesthetics. It is likely that neither lipid or protein but the entire hydrated lipid-protein complex is involved.

Next we must look at inter-relationships between the action of divalent calcium and local anaesthetics. There is considerable evidence that membrane bound calcium is dissociated from electrically excitable membranes when these are depolarized and that calcium bound in the membrane is necessary

for the initiation of the action potential [21]. There appears to be an interaction between sodium and calcium in the membrane structure. Many of the
effects of increasing external calcium are similar to those of local anaesthetics. In fact high external calcium concentrations antagonize local anaesthetic
action [22]. In the resting state of nerve the conductance channels for sodium
and potassium are likely blocked by calcium ion bridges neutralizing the
fixed negative charges within the membrane. Studies utilizing the calcium
[45] radioactive isotope have shown an increased uptake and release of
calcium with electrical stimulation or depolarizing drugs. Local anaesthetics
prevent this release of calcium. The view of TASAKI is that the active axon
membrane is a cation-selective membrane with a fixed charge capable of
two stable states determined by monovalent and divalent cation interactions,
and the configuration of the action potential is a reflexion of the rate of
exchange between univalent sodium and divalent calcium at the negative
sites in the membrane [23, 24].

Recent investigations on the excitation-contraction coupling mechanism
of muscle are pertinent here [25–31]. Depolarization conducted down the
central tubule of the triad, which is open to the outside of the muscle fibre,
releases calcium from the triad sacs which then reacts in turn with actin,
myosin and ATP to cause contraction. During relaxation the calcium
is strongly and actively rebound by elements of the sarcoplasmic reticulum.
In nerve this mechanism may not differ qualitatively from that in muscle. The
release of calcium on depolarization could activate the energy-producing
mechanism necessary to restore the membrane potential. Local anaesthetics
by preventing the calcium release and sodium influx would fix the membrane
in a non-depolarizable state and inhibit the excitation – recovery coupling
mechanism.

Of interest here are the studies of KUPERMAN and coworkers [32]. These
workers found that adenosine triphosphate and other nucleotides antagonized the effects of low calcium on isolated nerve. Further these nucleotides
antagonized the depressant action of procaine in low calcium but not cal-
cium-free Ringer. For example in nerves treated thirty minutes in 5×10^{-3} M
procaine and then in 1×10^{-2} M adenosine triphosphate, the action potential
returned to normal in one hour. Without the adenosine triphosphate treatment conduction did not return for two and a half hours. It was suggested
that calcium and adenosine triphosphate are somehow associated in the
membrane (compare with muscle!). Displacement of calcium by impulse
initiation releases membrane adenosine triphosphate with a resultant increase
in sodium permeability. Procaine and local anaesthetics in general may
interfere with this calcium-adenosine triphosphate association.

To conclude this preliminary discussion on basic actions of local anaesthetics the excellent studies of SKOU [33] on the activity of local anaesthetics on monomolecular films at an air-water interface must be mentioned.

At first Skou used films of stearic acid on water but later he used mono-layers of the mixed lipids from sciatic nerve. Interestingly he found that six local anaesthetics at approximately their minimal blocking concentrat-ions (Cm) increased the surface pressure of the mixed sciatic lipid mono-layers. It should be realized that the film or surface pressure is the difference in surface tension between a clean air-water surface and that of the surface covered with the spread films. The measurements can conviently be made with a Wilhelmy balance and force-area curves can thus be measured. The curves illustrated in Skou's studies clearly show that the local anaesthetics that are the most effective in increasing the surface pressure have the lowest minimal blocking concentrations. These minimal effective concentrations are dependent on pH; anaesthetic potency is greater at a high pH than at a low pH. Furthermore, the ability of local anaesthetics to increase the surface pressure in monolayers parallels the effect of pH on increasing the ability to block conduction. Skou's measurements showed that an average of 8.7×10^{13} local anaesthetic molecules were sorbed per square centimeter of lipid-water interface at the Cm and corresponded to an average change of 6.9 dynes per centimeter in surface pressure [see34]. Interestingly enough these figures are approximately the same for general anaesthetics at their minimal effective concentrations.

Interactions of amphiphilic molecules (defined as molecules which possess distinct regions of lipophilic and hydrophilic character) similar to those of local anaesthetics with mixed lipid monolayers (also amphiphilic) at an air-water interface may result in penetration of the monolayer [see 9]. The main effect of this penetration is an immediate rise in the surface pres-sure of the mixed film, a change in surface potential and the formation of a stable highly viscous mixed monolayer. If the amphiphile does not penetrate there is little change in the film characteristics. The fact that local anaesthe-tics do increase surface film pressure means that they must penetrate the mixed lipid monolayers. This suggests that a similar penetration probably occurs within the surface layers of natural membranes. Penetration of monolayers and for that matter biological membranes to form stable complexes within them depends primarily upon the establishment of strong interactions between the two amphiphiles i. e. the local anaesthetic and the mixed lipid monolayers or mixed lipid micelles in natural membranes. These interactions can be [1] polar, such as between lipid carboxyl groups and the dissociated cationic region of local anaesthetic molecules (ion-ion interaction) or the undissociated anaesthetic molecule (ion-dipole inter-action) or [2] non-polar such as interactions between the lipophilic segments of lipids and that of local anaesthetics. When both these interactions are satisfied the penetrating local anaesthetic molecule greatly increases the stability of monolayers with a consequent sharp rise in the surface pressure. It is important to note that only the polar interactions would be affected by pH. There is a considerable body of evidence which indicates that the tertiary amine is the anaesthetically active form [35–39], thus in local anaesthesia the polar membrane interactions are likely of the ion-dipole type. RITCHIE and GREENGARD however maintain that the active form is the cation [40]. It is of profound importance to the designer of more effective and less toxic local anaesthetics to appreciate the implications of these effects produced when amphiphilic molecules interact with membrane amphiphiles. For example the simple insertion of a double bond in the lipophilic segments of the molecule would greatly weaken the association between interacting amphiphiles. Variations in the properties of the polar groupings, proton activity and ionic strength of local anaesthetic molecules also would strongly affect the stability of interactions with surface films and biological membranes.

Although the tertiary amine is probably the most active form for anaesthesia it must not be thought that the cation form is not active on the membrane. In experiments on the transport of sodium from outside to inside in the frog's skin (measured by the current necessary to short-circuit the potential across the skin) it seems that local anaesthetics in the cation form increase sodium flux. For example at pH 7.8 procaine first increases the flux of sodium and then blocks, whereas at pH 6.0 there is no decrease in sodium flux. It should be remembered that LORENTE DE Nó found an enhancement of conduction followed by block in bullfrog A & C nerve fibres first bathed in a sodium deficient medium then treated with a local anaesthetic [41, 42]. Perhaps the depressant-convulsant activity of local anaesthetics on central nervous system synapses is related to these differential effects of the cation and tertiary amine on sodium conductance in the membrane. If increase in nerve membrane permeability to cations is dependent on neutralization of charge then it could only happen if the local anaesthetic was in the cationic form.

Chairman: Thank you Dr. WOLFE. I would like to ask Dr. TRUANT to relate what Dr. WOLFE has just been telling us to the action of local anaesthetics on nervous conduction, first of all in a single typical fibre, and then fibres of different size.

Truant: There are essentially three different sites at which local anaesthetics may come into contact with nerves under clinical conditions. The first and most peripheral is that following infiltration anaesthesia where the nerve structures and nerve endings have small diameters and are easily penetrated by local anaesthetic drugs. Secondly, in an increasing order of sensitivity, the unprotected spinal nerve roots in the subarachnoid space; and thirdly the nerve trunks in the epidural space or the long mixed nerves, where heavy connective tissue coverings create a formidable barrier to the penetration of local anaesthetics.

Now in considering the site of nerve blockade we must make a distinction between the generation of an action potential at a nerve ending, and the propagation of the signal along a nerve fibre. Lowenstein of New York has used the Pacinian corpuscle (which is in effect a pressure transducer) with its associated nerve fibre to illustrate the specific effect of local anaesthetics on impulse propagation as opposed to their generation of impulses [55].

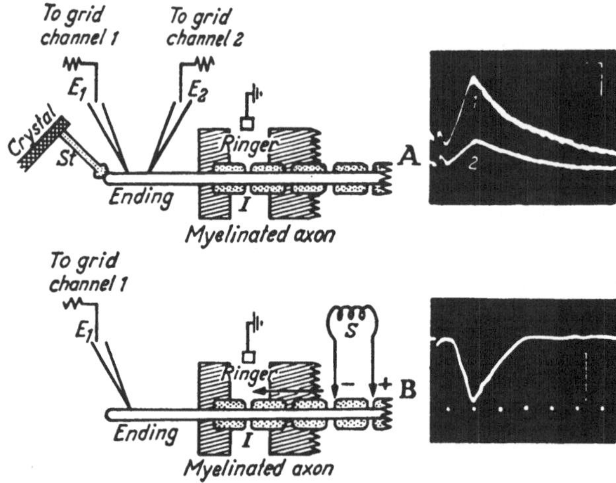

Fig. 1. Pacinian receptor. A. Electrotonic spread of current during crystal excitation. B. Electrical excitation of action potential in myelinated axon and propagation failure within the receptor ending. (Lowenstein, reference 55).

Fig. 1 shows a diagram of Lowensteins experimental design. A vibrating crystal excites the pressure-sensitive Pacinian corpuscle, and a generated signal (A) can be recorded from the corpuscle – this is the non-conducted or electrotonic action potential. If he retains the same intensity of vibration, but moves the recording electrode a small distance down the nerve a much smaller electrotonic potential is obtained, and this is not propagated beyond the first node of Ranvier (B). Now a very careful application of local anaesthetic between these two points does not affect the electrotonic potential, supporting the findings of others that local anaesthetics cannot affect the initial pressure-transducing event which generates the primary electrotonic potential. Blockade must therefore occur somewhere along the course of the nerve after the initial exciting current has become a propagated impulse.

Now let us proceed to examine the course of anaesthetic blockade on the propagated impulse in a single fibre. Fig. 2 shows a single motor fibre stimulated to produce a propagated impulse which can be recorded. Local anaesthetic is applied to the nerve between these two points and repeated stimuli are administered at intervals of one minute. The following effects can be seen:

1. Slowing of conduction.

2. Reduction in height of the propagated action potential.

3. Finally, in time, conduction blockade occurs when the action potential can no longer traverse the narcotized region.

However, if a stronger stimulus is applied we can once again obtain a propagated impulse across the partially narcotized region. Thus, local anaesthetics produce a graded depression and not an all-or-none effect.

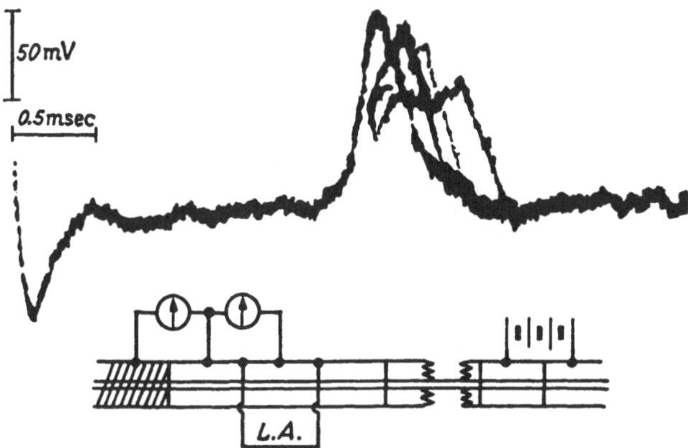

Fig. 2. Propagated action potential of a single nerve fibre (R. pipiens) during conduction block with Xylocaine hydrochloride 5 mM.

Moreover, the action potential decrements steadily as it passes along a segment of narcotized nerve, so that the degree of depression of a propagated impulse depends on the length of nerve affected by a local anaesthetic. These points have important clinical applications in regional anaesthetic techniques, and they may perhaps be seen even more clearly in another single fibre preparation, using a squid giant axon, in Fig. 3.

Conduction velocities can be measured between the points A and C and again you will notice the slowing in conduction, and lowering of the height of the action potential until finally complete block occurs in the narcotized area. However, it should be noted that if the depressed impulse has sufficient strength to pass the narcotized zone it immediately regains its normal stature on entering normal undepressed nerve.

Although there is an elevation in the threshold of excitability at the point of narcosis, the membrane potential remains normal as Dr. WOLFE has pointed out. Some investigators have shown that a small degree of hyperpolarization of the membrane may occur under certain exaggerated conditions, but this does not seem to be an important feature of the blocking process.

Thus there are four main events that occur during blockade: 1. The local action potential is reduced; 2. Conduction velocity slows; 3. There is a steady decrement of the action potential along the length of the narcotized segment, and 4. The membrane potential is unaltered.

During recovery the sequence of events of blockade is reversed.

Now, not all fibres are equally sensitive to the action of local anaesthetics. From time to time it has been stated that certain local anaesthetics are relatively more potent than others against so-called sensory fibres. But this is only a matter of concentration or degree; it is not a qualitative characteristic of any of the local anaesthetics. Differential blockade of the various diameters of fibre can only be obtained by changing the concentration that bathes them.

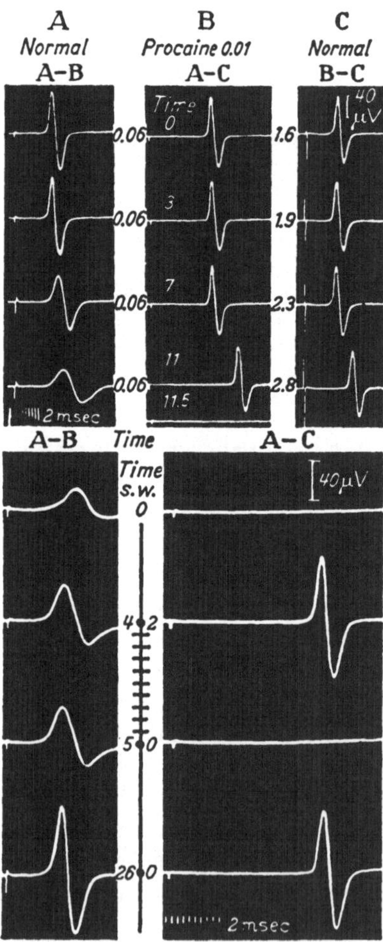

Fig. 3. Effects of procaine 10 mM superfusion on the bioelectric events of a stereoscopically prepared giant axon (2.8 cm) of the squid (Loligo). Stimulation, 1 per second; recordings were made from paraffin-isolated segments A, B, and C. Upper and lower oscillograms: blocking and recovery sequence, respectively. At hatched lines, superfusion was stopped and excess artificial sea water was removed.

In Fig. 4 we have a mixed nerve containing essentially three groups of fibres of different sizes. The largest fibres, which we refer to as the 'A' group can be excited by a relatively low intensity of current. The next largest, the 'B' group requires a current that is 5 or 10 times greater than the 'A' group, while the smallest, 'C' group requires a current of about 50–100 times greater than the 'A' group.

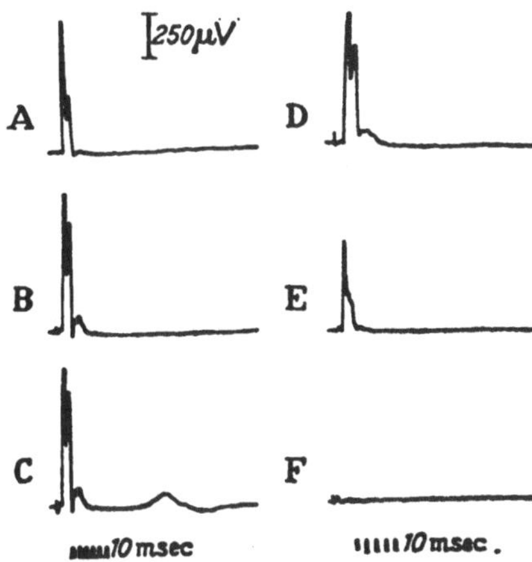

Fig. 4. Action potentials of bullfrog sciatic nerve (R. catesbiana) before and after application of procaine hydrochloride 20 mM. A, B, C, increase in current intensity; D, E, F, blocking sequence during a 10 minute period. (Mauro et al. Yale J. of Biology and Medicine 21, 113, 1964).

The 'A' fibres have a diameter of about 20 microns and conduct at the velocity of about 60 metres per second. The 'C' fibres have a diameter of less than 2 microns and conduct at about 2–4 metres per second.

Now, when local anaesthetics are applied to a segment of a mixed nerve, propagation ceases first in the relatively small fibres, as we all know, and in the recovery phase these are the last to regain conduction.

But differential blockade is not simply a question of fibre diameter, and there is considerable overlap of susceptibilities in the 'A' and 'B' fibres. Although most of the 'B' group are affected before most of the 'A' group, there are some fibres in the 'A' group with relatively large diameters that are blocked very early. There may be differences such as the degree of internodal distance to account for this.

It is usually stated that the dorsal or sensory nerve fibres are more susceptible than the ventral root fibres. But this statement is only partially true, for if you record from the dorsal and ventral roots at the same time you find that about 60 or 70% of the dorsal root fibres are still conducting when the ventral root begins to show marked evidence of blockade, and in both roots one sees a simultaneous reduction in all components of the compound spike. That is to say, some impairment of 'A', 'B' and 'C' fibres is going on concurrently. So the whole question of differential neural blockade with local anaesthetics is still a major problem that requires further investigation.

Section II.

Effects of local anaesthetics on contractile tissues

Chairman: Local anaesthetics affect not only nerve fibres but all types of excitable tissues, either directly or indirectly. Striated muscle fibres as well as the involuntary muscles of heart, blood vessels and uterus are all depressed by high blood levels of local anaesthetics, and death from overdosage is a cardiovascular death due to a combined fall of cardiac output and peripheral resistance with the heart and blood vessels inert and relaxed. Therefore it is important to consider the fundamental causes of this depression so that we can devise appropriate treatment in the event of accidents. We are concerned to know how much of this cardiovascular depression is due to a direct action on the muscle membrane and how much is an indirect mechanism due to impairment of catecholamine release from stores in muscle tissue.

Dr. Wolfe would you care to comment on this?

Wolfe: Given intravascularly local anaesthetics can cause a direct and intense cardiovascular depression. Even topical applications can produce a rapid rise in blood levels that can lead to cardiovascular depression. The depression probably is related to interference with cation fluxes across the muscle cell membrane just as in nerve. The mechanism of depression of impulse production and conduction in the heart by local anaesthetics is no different than in the nervous system. There have been reports [*see* 52] of an antagonism between xylocaine and adenosine triphosphate, the essential energy containing molecule for muscle activity, and also an activation of the activity of heart muscle adenosinetriphosphatase, an essential enzyme for muscle relaxation. However these properties are not found for all local anaesthetics.

As far as the effects of local anaesthetics on blood vessels are concerned I would like to make a few comments in connection with catecholamine release. This is quite a complicated and confusing area. There are two main views on the way in which norepinephrine is removed after release by sympathetic nerve stimulation. One maintains that norepinephrine is metabolically inactivated after combination with receptor in the effector area [44]. The other view is that the concentration of epinephrine reaching the receptor is controlled by the ability of nerve terminals to take up catecholaines [45]. There is truth in both theories. Now cocaine is unique among local anaesthetics in that it causes vasoconstriction; all the others are vasodilators and depress smooth muscle. What is the reason for this? It has been found that cocaine blocks the uptake of norepinephrine in sympathetically innervated organs thus potentiating its effect by permitting higher concentrations to reach the receptors [46, 47]. It also increases slightly the output of norepinephrine from splenic nerves but not splanchnic nerves. It is interesting that cocaine also significantly increases the effects of norepinephrine on increasing the plasma nonesterified fatty acid concentration [48]. Eliminating the hepatic circulation does not affect the potentiation. In some way cocaine interferes with the binding of norepinephrine by tissues. Of great interest is the finding that adenosine triphosphate is very probably the binding molecule for catecholamines in the adrenal medulla and probably all adrenergic nerve terminals [49–51]. Catecholamines are bound to adenosine triphosphate in the ratio of 4:1. Procedures which deplete tissue of catecholamines also deplete the adenosine triphosphate and the adenosine triphosphate recovery time course follows that of the increase in catecholamines. Thus in adrenergic nerve endings cocaine might antagonize the ability of adenosine triphosphate to take up catecholamines, thus potentiating the effects of these neurohumours. Postganglionic sympathetic denervation causes a drastic fall in norepinephrine content of sympathetically innervated organs and produces a maximal increase in sensitivity to exogenous norepinephrine. This sensitization is not further potentiated by cocaine.

There appears to be no general correlation between the potency of local anaesthetics and antagonism of various smooth muscle stimulators [*see* 53]. Actually this is an area that could well be studied. Further study of the effects of local anaesthetics on catecholamine release and storage and on specific catecholamine receptors is needed. As far as striated muscle is concerned local anaesthetics have a curare-like action. The chemical structure of procaine is not too dissimilar from acetylcholine. There is evidence that local anaesthetics compete with acetylcholine for the muscle receptor sites thus preventing the depolarizing action of acetylcholine. In fact a cell depolarized by ACh can be repolarized by a local anaesthetic such as tetracaine [54].

Chairman: Thank you Dr. WOLFE. In considering the cardiovascular hazards of local anaesthetics there is a tendency to take the facile view that neural and muscular effects go hand in hand, and that potency and toxicity are directly related. However, your remarks about the special features of cocaine suggest that perhaps other local anaesthetics may also have individual differences in their cardiovascular effects, so that the net result on all types of excitable tissues may not be the same. Dr. TRUANT have you any comments on this point?

Truant: I agree. Compounds that are equipotent as nerve blockers do not necessarily have the same degree of effect on the receptors in the myocardium and blood vessels. For example, HARRISON and his colleagues have

shown that procaineamide has greater depressant effects on the myocardium
than lidocaine, although the former is less potent as a local anaesthetic and
as an anti-arrhythmic agent, as shown in Fig. 5.

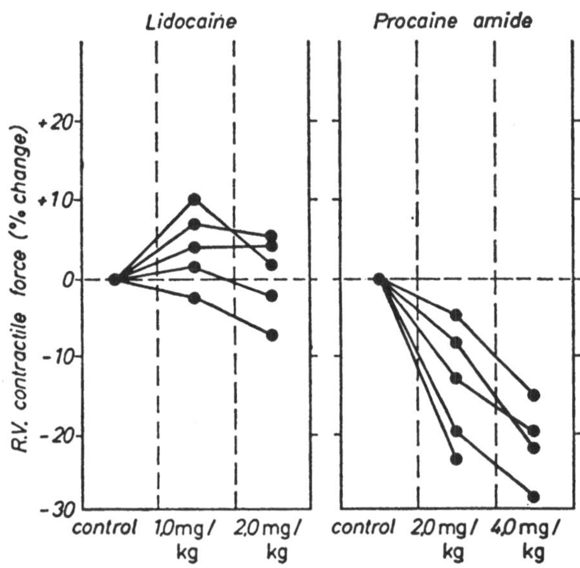

Fig. 5. Maximal changes in the contractile force of the right ventricle after the intravenous
administration of lidocaine or procaine amide. (Harrison et al. Circulation. **28**, 486, 1963).

Chairman: We will return to the question of smooth muscle depression
when we discuss toxicity.

Section III.

Molecular structure and design of local anaesthetics

Chairman: The precise nature of excitation in nerve and muscle is still
incompletely understood, and so it is unlikely that the perfect local anaesthetic will be designed until these processes are fully elucidated.

However, as Dr. WOLFE has pointed out, enough is now known about
the physical chemistry of excitable cell membranes to make a fair guess at
the sort of shape a good local anaesthetic molecule should have. But the
tailoring process is a lengthy and disappointing business, for while many
promising drugs may look well at first sight, further inspection usually
reveals that very few are sufficiently elegant to enter the small select group
that can withstand intense clinical scrutiny.

I would like the panel to discuss some of the broad principles of molecular configuration that determine the potency of local anaesthetics, and what
is more important, their toxicity.

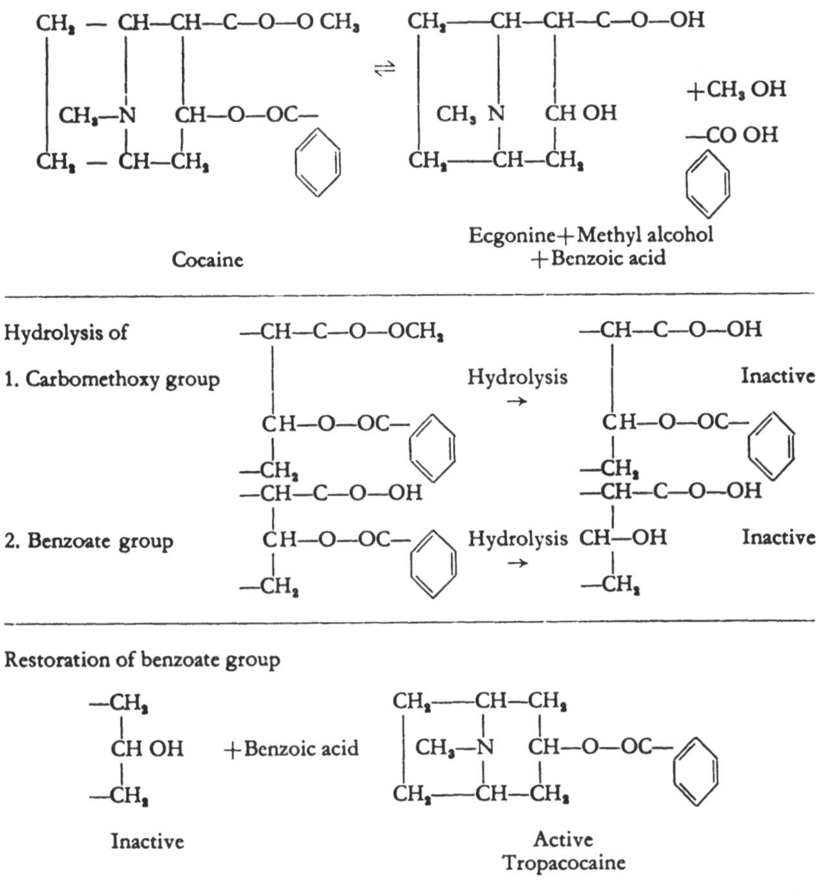

$$CH_2 - CH-CH-C-O-O\,CH_3 \quad\rightleftharpoons\quad CH_2---CH-CH-C-O-OH$$

Cocaine

Ecgonine+Methyl alcohol
+Benzoic acid

$+CH_3\,OH$

$-CO\,OH$

Hydrolysis of

1. Carbomethoxy group — $CH-C-O-OCH_3$ … Hydrolysis → $-CH-C-O-OH$ … Inactive

2. Benzoate group … Hydrolysis → … Inactive

Restoration of benzoate group

$+$Benzoic acid

Inactive

Active
Tropacocaine

Fig. 6

Geddes: Fig. 6 is intended to simplify the chemistry of local anaesthetics. Nature started off with a very complicated structure, namely cocaine. The synthetic chemist has simplified this by stripping away the non-essential parts after a process of elimination. First, hydrolysis of the carbomethoxy group caused loss of anaesthetic activity. Then hydrolysis of the benzoate group also gave loss of activity. But restoration of the benzoate group in a decarbomethoxylated compound was followed by restoration of local anaesthetic activity, and this compound was called tropacaine.

The next step was to demonstrate that the tropane ring was not essential. In Fig. 7 the potential procaine molecule lying within cocaine is indicated by the dotted line where the enclosed structural formula is to be found in the active part of cocaine. We can now see the simplicity of the procaine molecule. It is an ester derived from para-aminobenzoic acid. The ring of benzoic acid has lipophilic properties, while at the other end of the alkyl chain a tertiary amine group has hydrophilic properties.

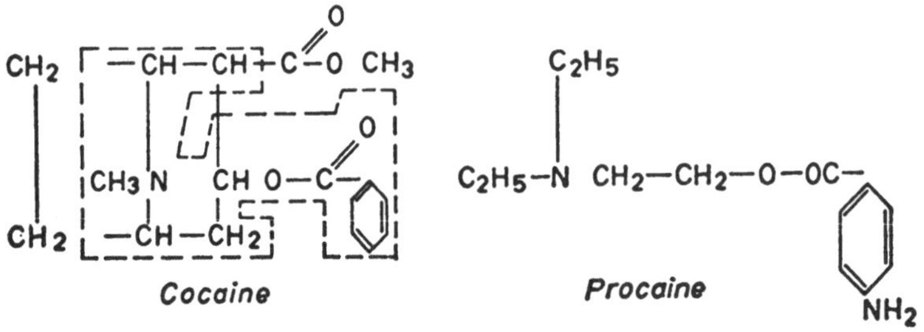

Fig. 7

In Fig. 8 we see representatives from two main groups of local anaesthetics, esters and amides. 2-chloroprocaine has been included for one reason only, and that is to show how a minor modification can cause quite a considerable alteration to the potency and speed of breakdown of a molecule. Chlorine attached to the 2-position of the para-aminobenzoic ring affects the stability of the neighbouring ester group. This allows enzymatic hydrolysis to proceed at a faster rate and also results in a lowering of the potency of 2-chloroprocaine compared to procaine [56].

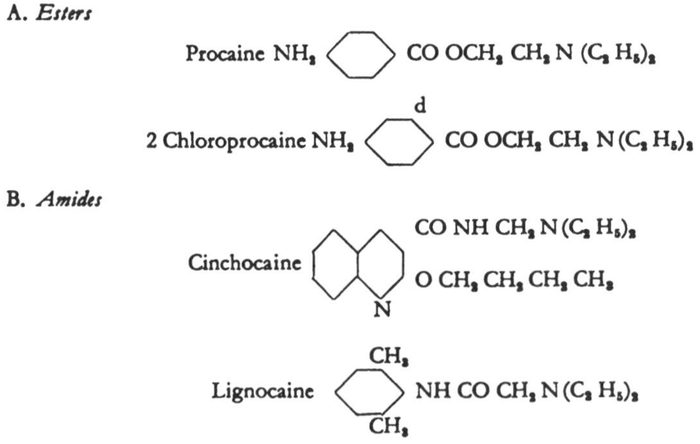

A. *Esters*

B. *Amides*

Fig. 8. Typical anaesthetic molecules.

Cinchocaine was the first of the drugs in the second group (the amides) to be used clinically [57]. Lignocaine was introduced by Lofgren [58], and was the archetype of a whole series of compounds having local anaesthetic activity, although very few of these are suitable for clinical use.

Fig. 9 shows one of the most recent drugs of this series, Citanest, compared to the formula for lignocaine. Both of these drugs are amides but they differ in some important respects. The two methyl groups on the ring of lignocaine are particularly interesting for they act to protect the amide bond from hydrolytic breakdown by stearic hindrance. In Citanest, on the other hand, the ring has lost one of its methyl groups, and the alkyl chain is different and ends with a secondary amine. Fig. 10 shows how methyl substitution in the benzene ring of similar compounds produces great alterations in their resistance to hydrolysis, depending on the spatial position of the methyl group [59]. Hydrolysis of the amide linkage is not affected

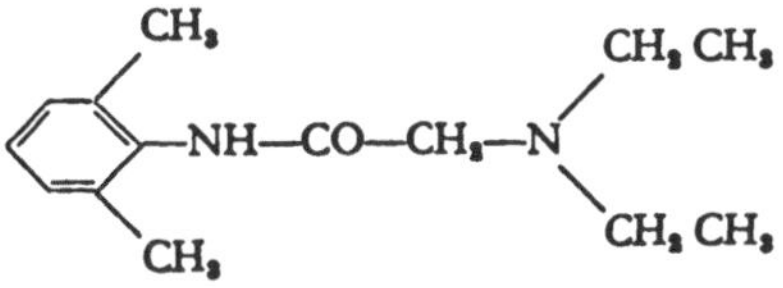

Lignocaine

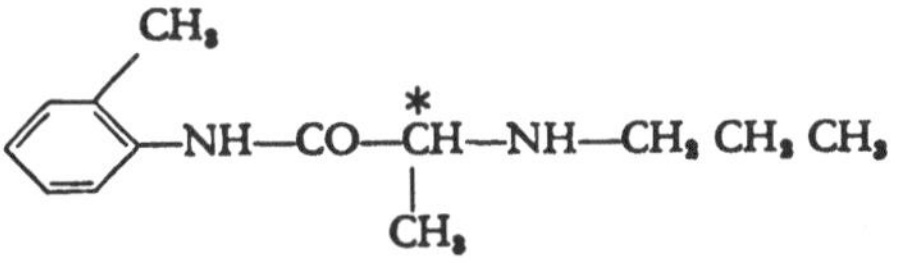

Fig. 9. Citanest.

	Time for 50 per cent hydrolysis in alkaline solution in hours
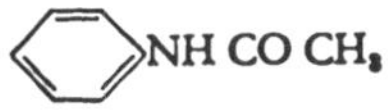 $\langle\ \rangle$NH CO CH$_3$	3 · 79
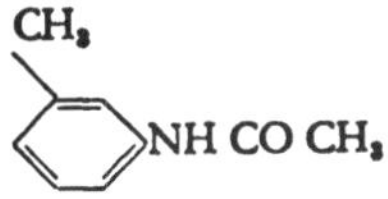 CH$_3$ $\langle\ \rangle$NH CO CH$_3$	3 · 89
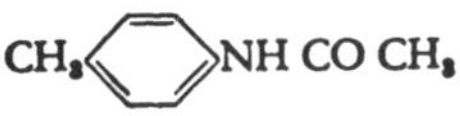 CH$_3$ $\langle\ \rangle$NH CO CH$_3$	3 · 9
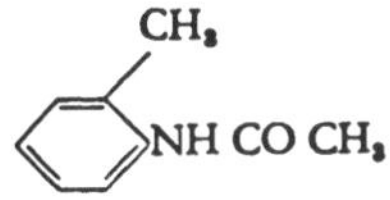 CH$_3$ $\langle\ \rangle$NH CO CH$_3$	17 · 16
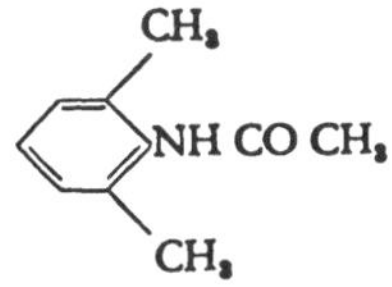 CH$_3$ $\langle\ \rangle$NH CO CH$_3$ CH$_3$	Very resistant

Fig. 10. Effect of methyl substitution.

when the methyl group is at a distance. But when the methyl group is close to the amide bond the splinting effect produces increased resistance to hydrolysis which is maximal when two methyl groups straddle the bond. From this it may be inferred that lignocaine is a more stable chemical than Citanest.

Chairman: Thank you Dr. GEDDES.

As anaesthetists we are continually being presented with newer types of local anaesthetics for clinical trial. Indeed, there is no limit to the number of these drugs that can be designed in the laboratory, but their clinical usefulness is determined by such things as their speed of onset, duration, and particularly their local and systemic toxicity.

However, just as a good horseman can pick a likely winner for a race by just glancing over the paddock, so the neurochemist can predict with fair accuracy how a drug will behave by an armchair study of its molecular structure. As an example Dr. WOLFE is unfamiliar with the new Swedish preparation LAC-43, and so I would like to ask him to analyze the structure of this drug for us, with a view to predicting its probable qualities as a local anaesthetic.

Wolfe:

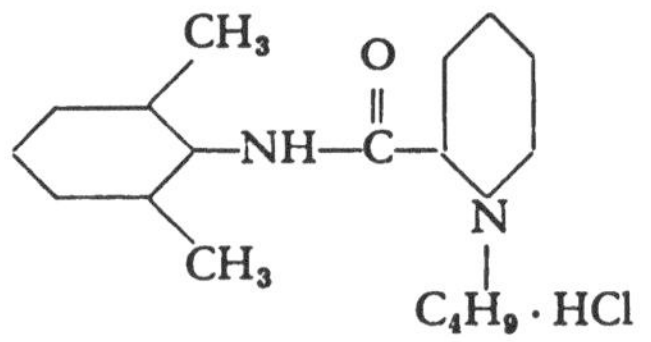

$$CH_3 \quad \overset{O}{\underset{\|}{}} $$

LAC-43

By just seeing this structure for the first time a number of its properties can be inferred. First of all it is an amide and thus would not be attacked or hydrolysed by esterases. This of course would prolong its biological activity. In the liver there are amidases which split this chemical linkage but their activity is very much less than the esterases. Another feature of this molecule is that it has a tertiary nitrogen in which one of the substituents is a butyl group. In contrast to the quaternary compounds tertiary amines can penetrate and dissolve in the lipid constituents of membranes. This property would probably increase the anaesthetic potency as well as the toxicity. The presence of a butyl stubstituent instead of a methyl would also be likely to increase toxicity since it is usual that toxicity increases when a homologous series is ascended (i.e. methyl to ethyl to butyl). The reason for this is probably due to the stronger and closer associations with which the longer aliphatic substituents can have with the aliphatic side chains of fatty acids in the membrane lipids. Another feature that can be inferred from this structure relates to its stability to enzymatic breakdown. This stability is not only related to the amide ester group but also to the absence of electrophilic substituents such as chlorine. Such substituents generally increase the potency and also the rate of degradation by tissue and plasma enzymes. Methaemoglobinaemia is one of the side effects of local anaesthetics that are rapidly absorbed in large quantities or given intravenously. This is usually brought about by a rapid increase in the blood levels of hydrolytic products such as acetanilide derivatives. I would suspect that LAC-43 would be unlikely to produce methaemoglobinaemia. In summary, this molecule is probably a potent, very long lasting local anaesthetic with minimal side effects, but it is also quite toxic – more so than xylocaine.

Chairman: Thank you Dr. WOLFE. Dr. TRUANT have you any comments on the subject of structure and design?

Truant: The question of potency and structure is extremely complex. Today the chemist is in a position to synthesize compounds which have sufficient lipophilic and hydrophilic characteristics to allow a fair prediction of their potency. But when it comes to predicting toxicity we are at a complete loss.

We have tried various approaches, particularly improving the ease with which local anaesthetics can be broken down to harmless residues in the body. As an example of this we have tried the esters, and the effect of chlorinating or hydroxylating in the 2-position of the benzene ring. These compounds are broken down very rapidly by pseudocholinesterase, as has been amply demonstrated by Dr. FOLDES in the case of 2-chloroprocaine [56]. We can also obtain similar effects with the amides.

The chief difference between the two main classes of compounds, the esters and the amides, lies in their rate of absorption. In general, the esters are hydrolyzed more rapidly, and are also absorbed more rapidly than the amides.

Section IV.

Uptake of local anaesthetics

Chairman: At this point we should turn our attention to the very important influence of pH and ionization on absorption, because so much of the uptake, distribution and excretion of local anaesthetics is determined not only by the intrinsic characteristics of a drug, but also by the hydrogen ion concentration of its solution and of the tissues into which it is injected.

Local anaesthetics are lipoid soluble bases that penetrate lipo-protein cell membranes as the non-ionized form. But unfortunately the non-ionized bases are insoluble in water, so that they have to be converted to water-soluble ionized salts before they can be injected. Thus we have a dilemma in the choice of solubilities in two incompatible phases, which can only be resolved by dynamic compromise, and a good local anaesthetic, like a politician, must be able to sit squarely on the fence, ready to move freely in either direction when occasion demands. The fence that these drugs have to sit on is the physiological range of pH, and a successful drug must have its point of balance, or ionization constant, as close to this range as possible.

The pharmacologists have been aware of this for many years, but clinicians have been slow to take advantage of this knowledge and to manipulate the pH of solutions and tissues as effectively as they might.

Dr. TRUANT would you care to enlarge on this matter before we go any further?

Truant: pH determines the rate at which any one of these local anaesthetic compounds will move across into the cell. At low pH there is a very high degree of ionization, while at high pH relatively large amounts of the base are present in the non-ionized form as in Fig. 11.

(High pH, Alkaline)

$$R \equiv N \cdot H^+ \; \xrightleftharpoons{\hspace{3cm}} \; R \equiv N + H^+$$

(Low pH, Acid)

Fig. 11. pH of solution and ionization of local anaesthetic base.

It is the non-ionized form that penetrates the electrical charges on the cell surface and travels across the membrane. However, in passing, I would like to emphasize that if you quaternarize a compound, and that entails putting a charge on it, the drug can still travel across a cell membrane, albeit at a slower rate.

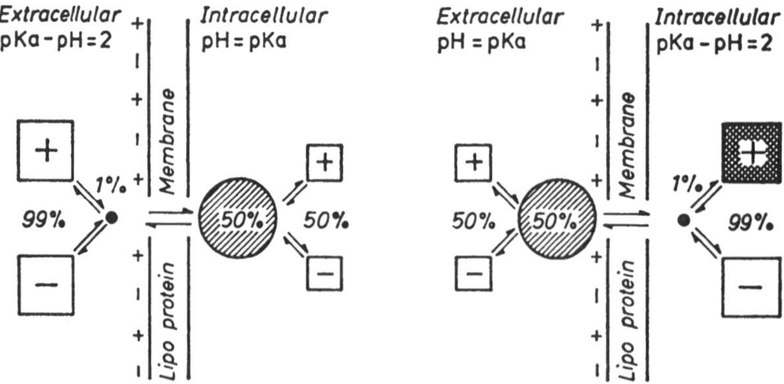

Fig. 12. Cellular uptake of local anaesthetics. Effects of pH and ionization constant (pKa). Non-ionized uncharged moiety of local anaesthetic base ●. Extracellular and intracellular local anaesthetic cation (charged) ○.

In Fig. 12 we see the effects of intra and extracellular pH on drug uptake. On the left we see the situation where a relatively acid solution is outside a cell of normal pH. The solution is highly ionized, relatively little drug is present as undissociated base, so that it moves very slowly and in small amounts into the cell. In the right hand part of the diagram the opposite state of affairs obtains. The external pH is high relative to the inside of the cell, and the extracellular pH equals the pKa of the drug, so that half of the drug is present as undissociated base, and now the drug passes into the cell much more rapidly. Once inside it becomes ionized by the intracellular acidosis and tends to remain sequestered in the cell.

Now there is a curious constancy in the amount of any given local anaesthetic drug that penetrates the axoplasm of a nerve. If varying strengths of procaine are applied to the external surface, say 5, 10, 15, or 20 millimolar, the time required to produce conduction blockade shortens from 17 minutes to 2 minutes with increasing concentration. However the amount found in the axoplasm is constant at about 4.2 millimoles (or roughly 100 micrograms for every 100 milligrams of wet tissue) regardless of the external concentration. A local anaesthetic that is two or three times as potent as procaine will have about half as much drug in the axoplasm at the time of conduction block.

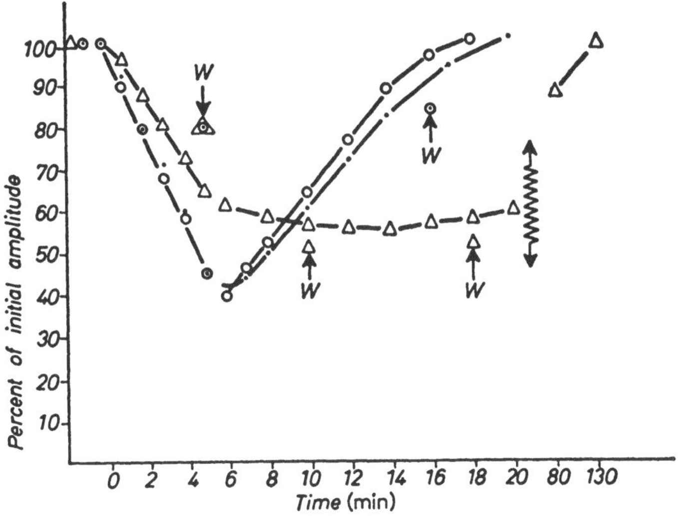

Fig. 13. Kinetic block and recovery of monophasic A spike fo frog sciatic nerve (R. pipiens) with procaine 20 mM • — • — •, Lidocaine 5 mM o – o – o and tetracaine 0.8 mM △ – △ – △. Ringer solution (w) pH 7.30 at 22° C. (Ref. Truant, A. P. and Takman, B. Differential physical-chemical and neuropharmacologic properties of local anesthetic agents. Anes. and Anal. **38**: 478-484, 1959).

All anaesthetics do not have similar kinetic characteristics. That is, their conduction blockade does not recede at the same rate. Fig. 13 illustrates this by a comparison of the blocking characteristics of procaine, lidocaine and tetracaine. Twenty millimoles of procaine are required to produce a 50% conduction block in a mixed nerve, whereas only one-quarter of this concentration of lidocaine is required to obtain the same degree of block. But, despite their different potencies the recovery pattern is the same for both compounds.

Chairman: Thank you Dr. TRUANT. For some time now a number of researchers have been looking into the effects of carbon dioxide on intracellular pH. Carbondi oxide is an interesting material, since it is formed by biological processes and at the same time is essential to them in a fairly narrow range of concentrations [60]. It also has the property of passing across cell membranes with great rapidity, lowering intracellular pH and producing a change in degree of polarization of the cell membrane [61, 62].

These properties are of considerable interest from the practical standpoint of augmenting anaesthetic blockade. A low intracellular pH should attract more anaesthetic base into the cells, and an altered membrane potential will diminish the efficiency of excitable tissues.

Dr. TRUANT, I know you have been doing some work on the potentiating effects of CO_2 and local anaesthetics in isolated nerves. I wonder if you would tell us a little about this work.

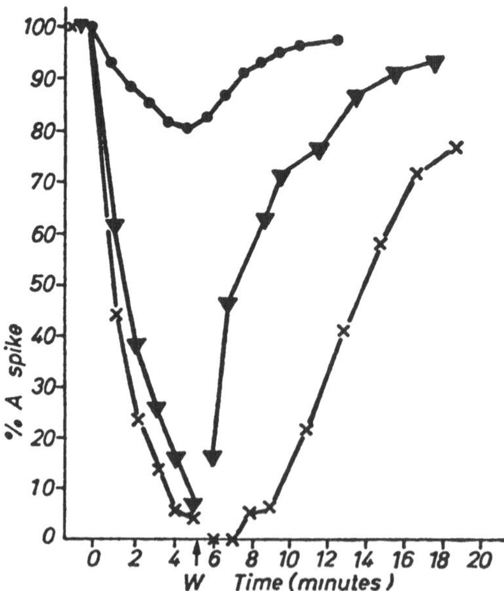

Fig. 14. Effect of Lidocaine HCl 1 mM ● – ●, 10 mM △ – △, 1 mM lidocaine equilibrated with 10% CO_2 x — x, on monophasic A spike in the sciatic nerve (1.8 cm length) of the frog (R. pipiens) – Ringer solution (w), pH 6.89 at 22° C.

Truant: Yes, the work was done on frog nerves. In Fig. 14 we see that one millimole of lidocaine at pH 6.89 produces about 20% block. In order to have a complete block we need 10 millimoles. However, if we add 10% carbon dioxide to the 1 millimolar solution we obtain a complete block – that is at one-tenth of the concentration that was necessary in the absence of carbon dioxide. This increased activity appears to be due to increased uptake of local anaesthetic by the nerve.

Of course "in vivo" neural uptake can also be increased by the use of a vasoconstrictor such as epinephrine. Hyaluronidase has also been advocated for the same purpose. However, hyaluronidase does not increase uptake, it only increases the lateral dispersion of the drug, so actually the nerves pick up less.

Chairman: Thank you Dr. TRUANT. Clinical experience confirms that vasoconstrictors do increase tissue uptake by preventing blood-stream absorption (and perhaps also by decreasing local tissue pH) whereas hyaluronidase increases the surface area for blood-stream absorption and so reduces the amount available for local uptake and nerves.

I would like to confirm Dr. TRUANT's in vitro findings with carbon dioxide and conduction blockade. Apart from the properties of carbon dioxide that we have mentioned, it is of course also an acid, and so can combine with local anaesthetic bases to form soluble salts. Two years ago, at Dr. TRUANT's suggestion, and with the help of the Astra Research Laboratories at Worcester, Massachusetts, we did some in vivo experiments using anaesthetic solutions made of the local anaesthetic bases combined with carbon dioxide at a pCO_2 of 700 mmHg. These solutions have since shown great promise clinically in several hundred cases of epidural block. These CO_2-base solutions have a short latency of onset, and their quality of analgesia and the intensity of motor block is superior to that of their orthodox hydrochloride counterparts [63]. Being bottled in ampoules with carbon dioxide at atmospheric pressure they give a gratifying sound when opened in a warm room, and their sparkling appearance has given them the nickname of "champagne".

These solutions exemplify a trend in local anaesthesia which I think will become more pronounced. The local anaesthetic bases available today are very effective, and it is unlikely that a pharmacological breakthrough will provide any notably superior drug. The technical limits of effectiveness are within the tissues, and the tissue barriers themselves, and we must find safe and acceptable ways to manipulate neural susceptibility, and to increase the speed of tissue uptake. A high pCO_2 in the vicinity of the local anaesthetic is one way of doing this.

Dr. GEDDES, have you anything to add to this?

Geddes: The effect of pH on the absorption of local anesthetics is not really a new discovery – at least it has been known empirically by the inhabitants of Peru for many centuries. Fig. 15 shows some of the equipmend used by the Andean Indians to alkalinize their saliva. The poporo or gourds contain the alkali which is made by burning shells or limestone, and the resulting llipta, as it is called, is mixed with coca leaves to aid extraction and absorption of cocaine.

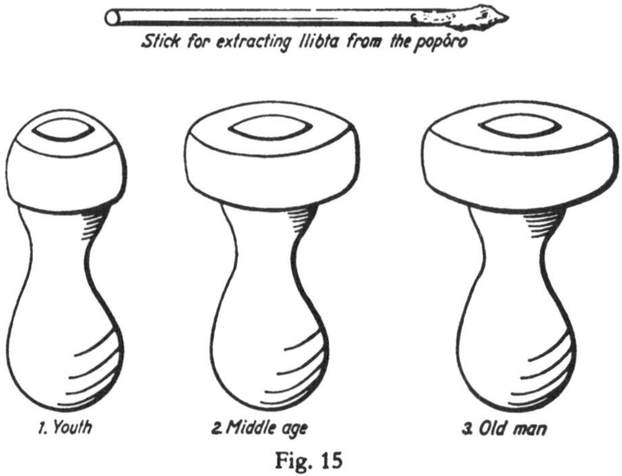

Fig. 15

Chairman: Alterations in sensitivity to local anaesthetics occur with age, so that the drugs appear not to be uniformly potent throughout the normal life span. The clinical anaesthetist should be aware of the effects of ageing if he wishes to be precise in his dosage. Moreover, from the investigational point of view it is important to bear in mind the effects of age when comparing the relative potencies of two or more drugs in different groups of patients.

Eriksson: When studying the duration of Citanest in fingerblocks I was quite surprised to find that the duration of the finger-blocks was much longer in old subjects than it was in the young ones [64]. Fig. 16 shows that there is a correlation between age and duration. First it was a little difficult to explain this, but from other experiments I know that the degree of the vascular supply at the site of injection is very important for the duration of the block. If I make an intracutaneous wheal with a weak local anaesthetic solution (Table 6), I can do that over and over again, and get a duration of 6–7 minutes. If the blood circulation is shut off by a tourniquet I prolong the duration of the wheal for almost the same time that circulation is occluded. We all know that old people don't have as good a peripheral circulation as young people have, and this is one possible explanation of the difference. It has also been shown by a group of researchers in Boston that the pH of tissues in old people is lower than in young people. So, once again, we may come back to the fact that it may be the problem of pH that is the explanation. I think however that the chairman also has another explanation.

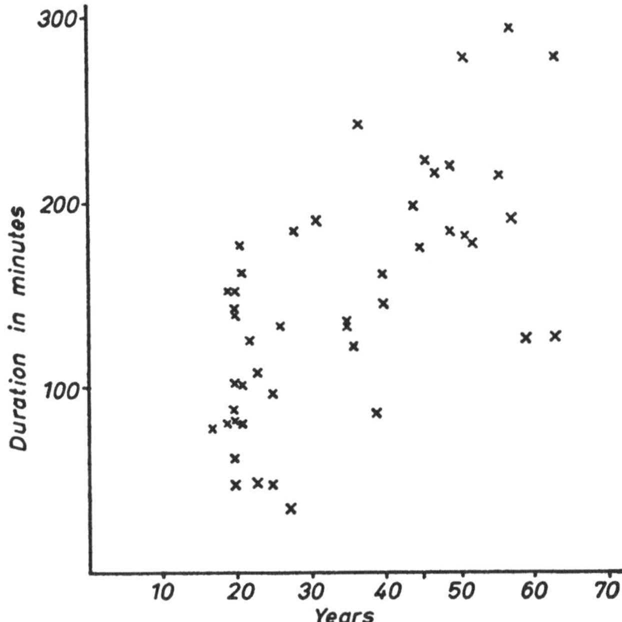

Fig. 16. Age duration of finger-blocks with Citanest. Distribution of corresponding values of age and duration of anaesthesia for L[67]. Mean duration for patients, age < 40 yrs: 110 min, > 50 yrs: 207 min.

Table 6. *Duration of anaesthesia in intracutaneous wheals in intact and ischaemic skin. Ischaemia was produced by stasis for 30 minutes*

Preparation	Conc.	Mean durations*			Difference	
		Without stasis	Stasis under 30 min.	Time of stasis subtracted	Mean**	Range
Xylocaine		7.0	36.2	6.2	0.8	−1 to 3
L 67	0.04 %	7.2	33.2	3.2	4.0	1 to 8
Carbocaine		5.6	33.6	3.6	2.0	−1 to 6
Xylocaine		15.1	40.1	10.1	3.8	−6 to 16
L 67	0.30 %	13.6	41.9	11.9	1.7	−8 to 11
Carbocaine		15.9	41.6	11.9	4.3	−5 to 16

    * Minutes.

    ** The mean of the differences was calculated from the differences of each paired observation.

114 P. R. Bromage

Chairman: The relation of age to potency of local anaesthetics is not surprising when we consider other aspects of ageing, for most of our physiological functions decline steadily with age. Fig. 17 shows three typical age-dependent curves to remind you of this. First, the number of myelinated fibres in a nerve root, second the conduction velocity in peripheral nerves, and third the capillary resistance of the skin. One could substitute many other biometric data, and they would all fall along a similar ageing curve.

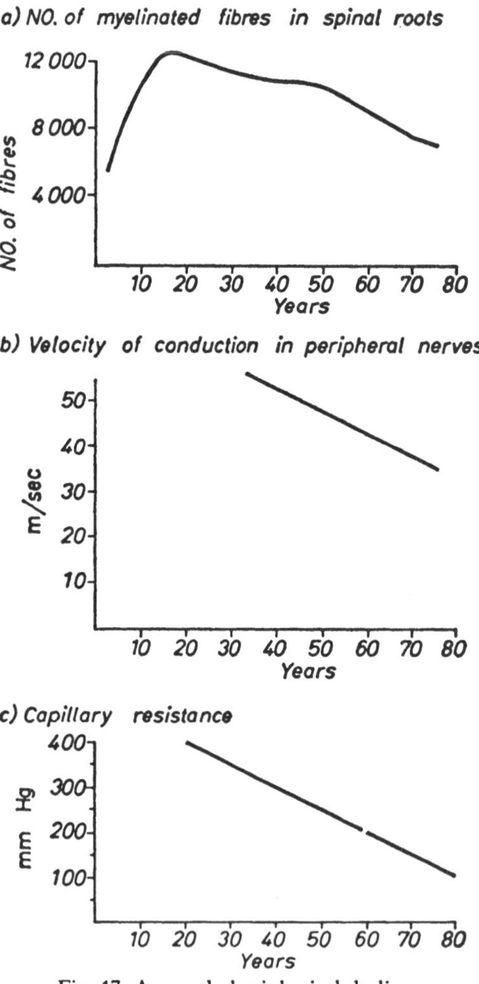

Fig. 17. Age and physiological decline.

When we superimpose the effects of a local anaesthetic upon such a pattern of biological change we may expect to find similar age-dependent relationships. And we should not forget that we are considering biological age rather than chronological age. The saying that a man is as old as his arteries is well illustrated by the segmental spread of analgesia in epidural blockade. Normally, young adults in their early twenties require two or three times more drug than an octogenarian to block a given number of spinal segments, and the decline in dose requirements is almost linear between these ages (Fig. 18).

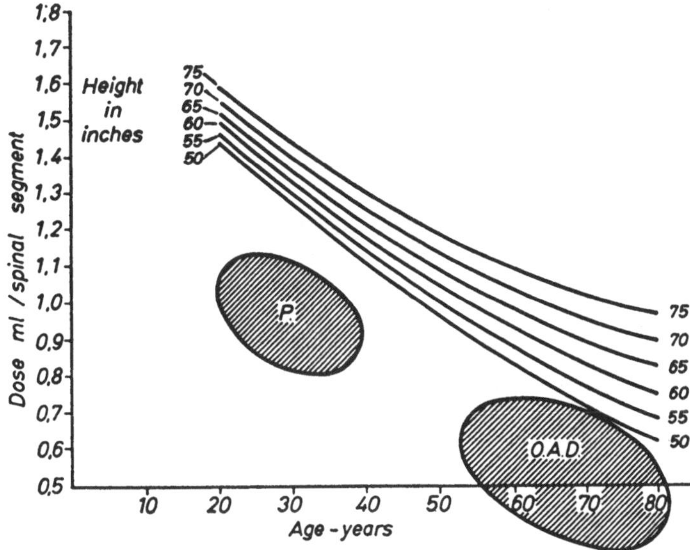

Fig. 18. Effects of age on epidural dose-requirements, and modifications produced by pregnancy (P) and occlusive arterial disease (OAD).

However, patients with occlusive arterial disease (OAD) from arteriosclerosis or diabetic angiopathy behave as if they were very much older than their years, and dose-requirements are reduced in proportion to the severity of the disease [65]. Pregnancy (P) also mimics a temporary physiological ageing in the pattern of response to subarachnoid or epidural blockade [66].

These differences are very important from a practical point of view, and ignorance of them may lead the anaesthetist to administer dangerous or even lethal overdoses to susceptible patients. The underlying cause of these age differences is still obscure, but it is probably a combination of several factors. It may be a question of tissue pH as Dr. ERIKSSON suggests, or it may be a deterioration of the quantity and quality of the conducting elements and the tissue barriers around them. In pregnancy hormonal as well as mechanical factors are obviously involved.

Section V.

Elimination of local anaesthetics

Chairman: This section will open the way to a discussion of toxicity of local anaesthetics because we must consider toxicity in terms of the balance between uptake and elimination, and the resulting concentration in the tissues at any given time.

Slow elimination is likely to be associated with higher tissue levels and greater toxicity than when a drug is rapidly broken down and excreted. We should therefore consider not only the drugs themselves and their susceptibility to excretion, but also the body's mechanisms of excretion and the ways in which these may be rendered more efficient.

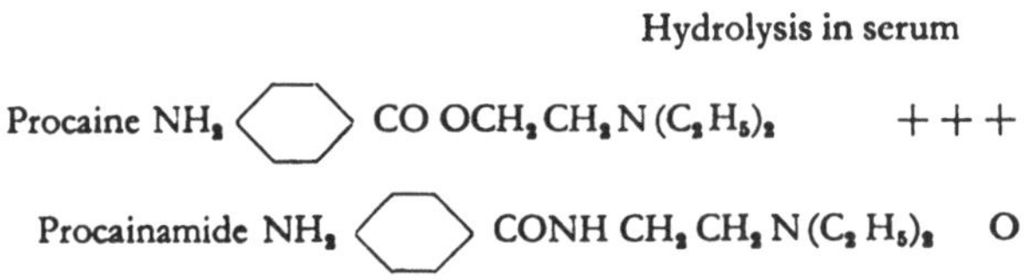

Hydrolysis in serum
Procaine NH_2 CO $OCH_2CH_2N(C_2H_5)_2$ +++
Procainamide NH_2 CONH $CH_2CH_2N(C_2H_5)_2$ O

Fig. 19. Effect of amide linkage.

Xylocaine
CH_3
NHCO CH_2 N C_2H_5 C_2H_5
CH_3
Oxidation
Oxidation
Hydrolysis
Conjugation
Decarboxylation
Urine
Bile
$C^{14}O_2$

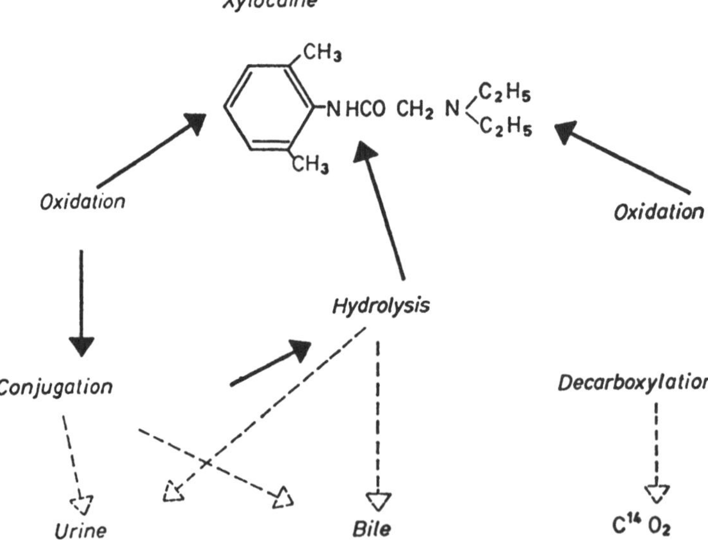

Fig. 20. Breakdown of lignocaine in the body.

Geddes: As I mentioned earlier the linkages of the ester and amide groups of local anaesthetics are very important, not only for their clinical stability but also for their susceptibility to enzymes in the body. The ester group in procaine is readily hydrolized (Fig. 19), not only in serum, but in nervous tissue, and especially in the liver. However, as Dr. WOLFE has previously mentioned, a completely different enzyme system is necessary when an amide linkage is present. Fig. 20 shows a summary of the possible points of attack for the breakdown and excretion of lignocaine. Apart from hydrolysis of the amide group, which has been shown to occur [67], lignocaine can also be oxidized in the 4-position of the benzene ring [68]. Once an OH group has been introduced in this position conjugation is possible. Conjugation may then be followed by excretion as an ethereal sulphate in the urine, or by hydrolysis to other breakdown products.

The molecule can also be attacked at the opposite end, and HOLLUNGER in Sweden has shown that oxidation of one of the ethyl groups can occur [69]. After administration of C^{14} labelled lignocaine some $C^{14}O_2$ can ultimately be traced, indicating that there is a complete metabolism of the labelled part of the molecule [67], but the main pathway of excretion of metabolites is in the urine.

In the rat, cannulation of the bile duct and chromatography and autoradiography of the bile have shown that numerous metabolites of lignocaine are excreted in the bile. It is not known whether these products are reabsorbed by the gastrointestinal tract and then re-excreted.

It appears that lignocaine can only be broken down at one site in the body, namely the liver, but Citanest is also degraded by kidney slices, in vitro [70].

Table 7. *Renal clearance studies of citanest and xylocaine.*

	Citanest (5 cases)		Xylocain (6 cases)	
Prime dose mg/kg	1.41	(1.19–1.79)	1.58	(1.35–2.0)
Infusion μg/kg/min	61.1	(53.6–80.4)	54.9	(35.1–68.2)
Total I.V.	442	(427–609)	523	(382–663)
$P_{CiT. S. XYL.}$	1.3	(0.9–1.7)	2.3	(1.4–3.0)
C_{IN} ml/min/1.73 m²	104	(86–143)	119	(95–143)
$C_{PAH,}$ ml/min/1.73 m²	581	(417–787)	614	(439–746)
C_X/C_{IN}	2.4	(1.2–3.6)	0.8	(0.2–2.6)

Mean values and ranges from five cases given Citanest and six cases given Xyclocaine. The experiments were performed together with inulin and PAH clearances, and these showed normal values, indicating normal renal hemodynamics. The mean of $C_{Citanest}/C_{IN}$ is 2.4 indicating a tubular secretion of Citanest. The mean of $C_{Xylocaine}/C_{IN}$ is 0.8 suggesting tubular reabsorption. Note the wide ranges.

Thus the complete mechanism for eliminating these local anaesthetics is not simple.

Eriksson: As little is known about the renal excretion of local anaesthetics, Granberg and I have tried to study the renal clearance of two local anaesthetics, lignocaine and Citanest [71]. We did this in volunteers and patients without any known renal disturbance or renal disease. Lignocaine or Citanest was added to inulin and PAH, during normal renal clearance studies. After a priming dose we injected the substances by means of a constant-speed syringe pump, and determined the concentrations of the substances in blood and urine. Table 7 shows that we got normal clearance for inulin and PAH, indicating normal haemodynamic conditions. The mean of the ratio clearance for Citanest, over clearance for inulin $^{C}Cit/^{C}IN$ was found to be 2.4. This indicates that besides a glomerular filtration of Citanest, there must also be a tubular excretion – while for lignocaine, $^{C}Lig^{C}IN$ is

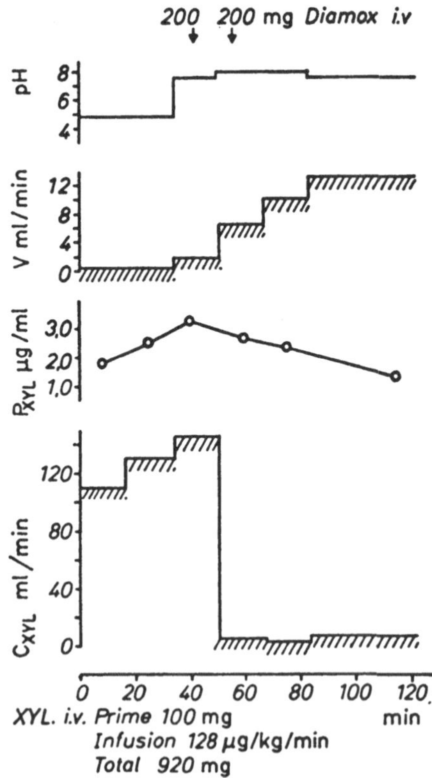

Fig. 21. The effect of alkalinisation of the urine on the Xylocaine clearance. The subject had taken NH₄Cl tablets the day before the investigation which gave the urine a pH of 4.8 400 mg Diamox (carbonic anhydrase inhibitor) intravenously raised the pH of the urine to 8.0. In spite of a twenty-fold increase of the urine flow, there was a forty-fold decrease of the Xylocaine clearance.

0.8, indicating that there must be a tubular reabsorption of lignocaine. Lignocaine and Citanest are weak bases, and according to MILNE and his co-workers [72], weak bases and weak acids can be excreted via the kidney by non-ionic diffusion as well as the usual glomerular filtration and tubular excretion. Non-ionic diffusion or passive tubular secretion implies transfer of material down an electrochemical gradient. Energy is only expended indirectly for the establishment of the gradient down which passive diffusion occurs. In acid urine, the equilibrium between ionized and non-ionized local anaesthetic is shifted in favour of the charged form, since hydrogen ions bind free base. Non-ionic diffusion is possible as the freely-diffusible base (which has been diffused from the plasma) is rapidly converted into the non-diffusible cation in the acid urine. The non-ionic diffusion thus depends on the pH of the urine, and on the urine flow. Fig. 21 shows an experiment where the pH of the urine of a volunter was shifted from acid to alkaline. The volunteer was given ammonium-chloride the day before the experiment, resulting in a low pH of the urine and a rather high clearance. But when we gave him 400mg of Diamox ^{R}, the pH of the urine rose, while the clearance of lignocaine fell tremendously, as much as forty-fold. Fig. 22, showing some similar cases, once again stresses the great importance of pH in the transfer of local anaesthetics across cellular boundaries.

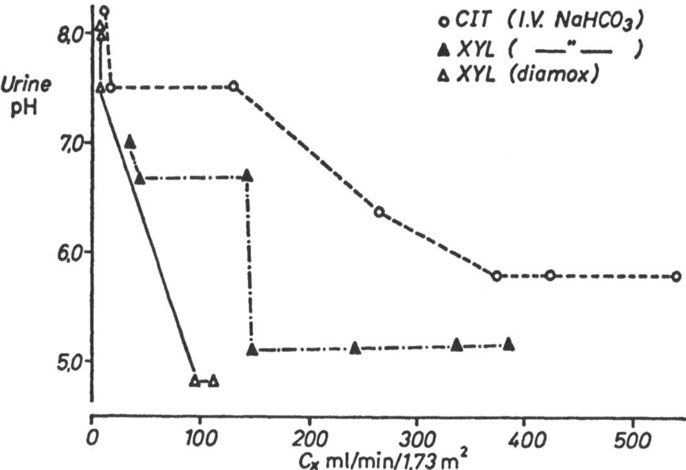

Fig. 22. Effect of urine pH on the clearances of Citanest and Xylocaine. Results from three investigations. In all cases the clearance decreased markedly as the urine was alkalinised by intravenous NaHCO₃ or Diamox.

Chairman: We tend to think of pH in terms of the most commonly measured fluid, arterial blood. Thank you Dr. ERIKSSON for reminding us of the importance of hydrogen ion concentration in other body fluids and in other body compartments, and its relation to the excretion of lipoid-soluble bases. Hydrogen ion concentration can be altered over quite a wide range in a controlled regional manner by intelligent manipulation of respiratory and electrolyte exchange.

Section VI.

Toxicity of local anaesthetics

Chairman: A vast number of local anaesthetic drugs have been investigated by pharmaceutical researchers, but very few possess the essential clinical requirements of low toxicity and high anaesthetic potency. Toxicity may be local due to tissue irritation at the site of injection, or due to systemic effects after absorption into the blood stream. We will only consider the latter in our present discussion.

As pointed out earlier, local anaesthetics depress *all* excitable tissues, and so they have their effects on voluntary and involuntary muscle, as well as on nervous tissue. It is the depressant effects on cardivascular musculature that are most dangerous and cause death from overdosage. Unfortunately, the very qualities of a drug that produce high anaesthetic potency also tend to produce cardiovascular depression.

Truant: In passing, one should note that not all compounds that are equipotent as anaesthetics have a similar degree of depressant effect on the myocardium. Thus, in comparing lidocaine, procaine and procainamide, the latter two drugs depress the contractility of the human myocardium more than lidocaine, although they are less effective as local anaesthetics.

Usubiaga: We must be aware that any consideration dealing with systemic effects of local anaesthetics in man, necessarily involves two basic premises: first, man must be the subject of the experiments, and second, the intravenous route of administration is preferred. Differences in enzymatic activity prevent any comparison between the potency and toxicology of different local anaesthetic drugs in animals and man. The use of the intravenous route is necessary in experimentation because the systemic effects observed in clinical work, after the introduction of local anaesthetics, imply the previous passage of their molecules through the blood stream.

The distribution of local anaesthetics after intravenous administration takes place in three main ways: site of action, attachment to non-specific structures named acceptors, and lastly breakdown by enzymatic or non-enzymatic mechanisms. The process involved in the case of procaine is shown in Fig. 23. It is clear that the actual amount of local anaesthetic arriving at the central nervous system or other site of action, is not only influenced by the total dose, rate of injection and pH of the body, and blood perfusion of the tissue, but also by the activity of the splitting mechanisms and by the number and disposition of the non-specific acceptors or "sites of loss". Now, two ways of prolonging the drug's effect are enzymatic inhibition and drug displacement from non-specific carriers. Here, we will outline only the first one, that is enzymatic inhibition.

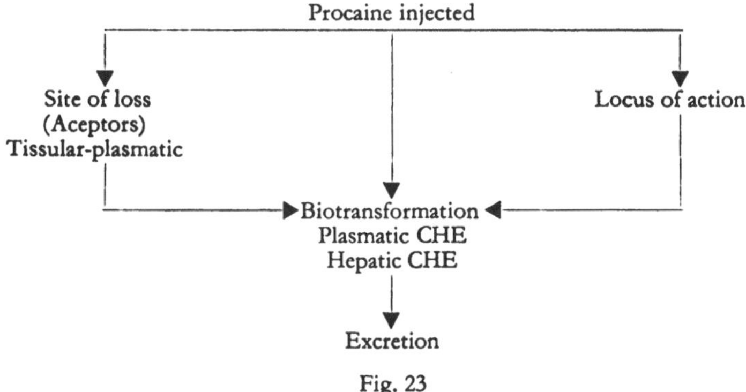

Fig. 23

Plasma cholinesterase may be inhibited reversibly or irreversibly by many substances. One of the reversible inhibitors used in clinical anaesthesia is hexaflorenium. We have demonstrated in man that the injection of hexaflorenium delays the breakdown of the procaine molecule and prolongs the length of systemic analgesia resulting from the intravenous injection of 10 mg per kg of procaine (Fig. 24). Whether or not this principle can be applied to prolong other effects produced by the ester-type of local anaesthetics, such as the anti-arrhythmic ones is now under study elsewhere.

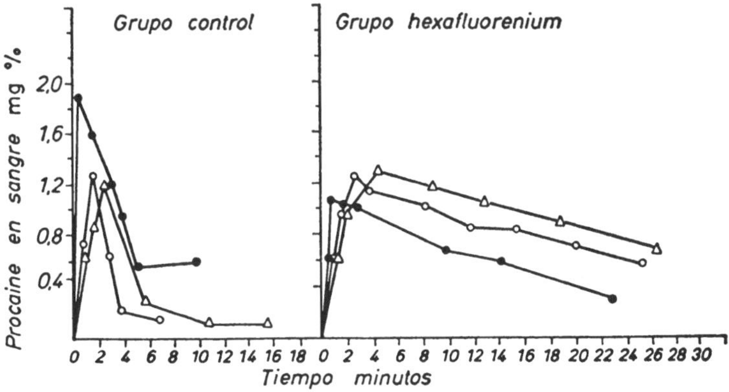

Fig. 24. Intravenous procaine. Persistence of high blood concentrations after hexaflorenium.

Another way of modifying the splitting capacity of pseudocholinesterase is by varying the concentration of the local anaesthetic substrate.
In Fig. 25 you can see the rate of breakdown of increasing amounts of
procaine in the presence of a fixed amount of the enzyme. The values for

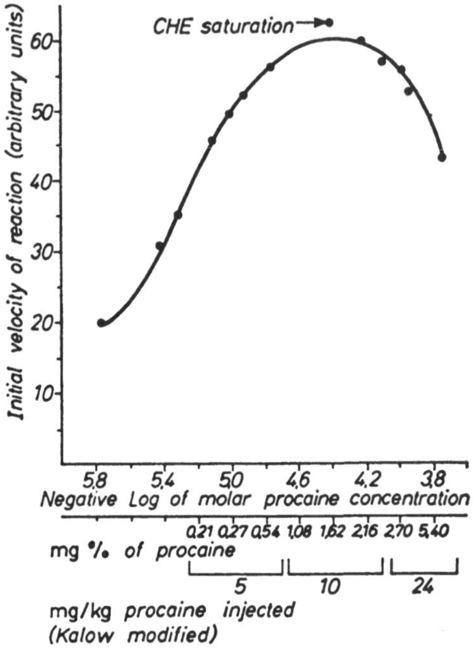

Fig. 25. Pseudocholinesterase and rate of procaine breakdown.

procaine are expressed in the first line of the horizontal axis as molar concentrations, in the second line as mg per 100 ml of plasma, and in the third
line as dose injected in mg per kg of body weight. Kalow has demonstrated
in vitro [73], that procaine concentrations over 10^{-4} M are able to saturate
plasma cholinesterase, diminishing the initial rate of biotransformation.
We have found similar plasma levels in man following the intravenous administration of 10 mg per kg of procaine.

The duration of apnea produced by a given dose of succinylcholine can
be prolonged by adminstering increasing amounts of local anaesthetics such
as procaine or lidocaine (Fig. 26). A slight prolongation of succinylcholine
apnea is produced by procaine in doses up to 10 mg/kg, and by lidocaine in
all doses. However, in doses over 10 mg/kg procaine provoked a marked
potentiation of the paralyzing effect of succinylcholine. Since inhibition of
pseudocholinesterase takes place with doses of procaine over 10 mg/kg we
must conclude that this is the cause of the sharp rise in the apnea curve for
procaine. As the anticholinesterase activity of lidocaine is very weak, the

first part of the curve may be explained on the basis of succinylcholine displacement from non-enzymatic sites, i. e. acceptors. The practical implication of this point is that the greater the plasma cholinesterase inhibitory effect of a local anaesthetic, the longer will be the length of apnea when succinylcholine and the local anaesthetic are administered together.

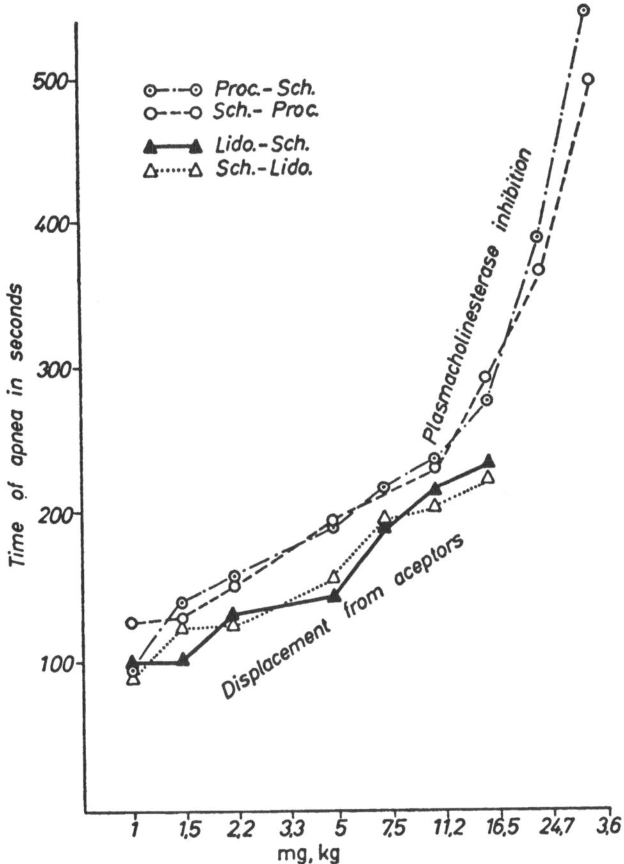

Fig. 26. Effect of increasing doses of procaine and lidocaine on duration of succinylcholine and apnea.

Geddes: I think it is most important while dwelling on the chemistry of local anaesthetic compounds to realize that the two main groups can be dealt with in the body in a different way. In the amide group it is not metabolism that is responsible for saving the individual from the acute toxic properties of these agents; it is essential to appreciate that it is redistribution, for metabolic processes are too slow to cope with an immediate overdose.

It is also important to appreciate that no toxic reactions' arise until a
threshold concentration of the drug is reached at the point where the
toxic action is to be engendered. Now, when you give these drugs the
quickest way of getting them into the body is to give them intravenously
and to illustrate this point I would like to show two figures from some
studies carried out by our Chairman [74]. Fig. 27 shows a patient who has
had two separate infusions of lignocaine, that is, one of the amide group of
local anaesthetics. Following the first injection there was no fall in blood
pressure despite an appreciable rise in the blood concentration of lignocaine.

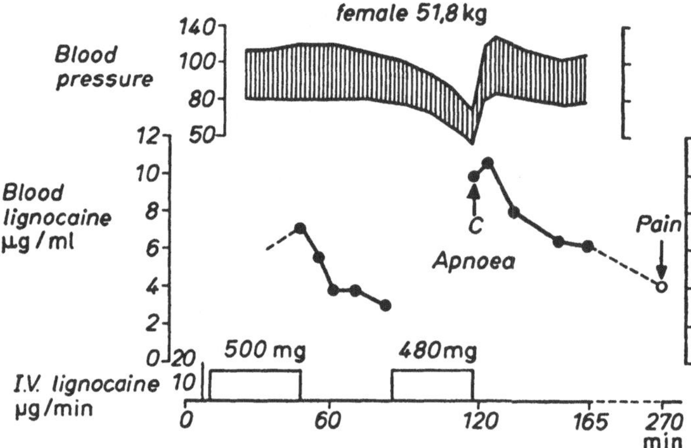

Fig. 27. Concentrations of lignocaine in the venous blood after intravenous infusion.
C = convulsion. At this point 100 mg of thiopentone were given to abort the convulsion,
followed by 10 mg of methylamphetamine to raise the blood pressure (Bromage and
Robson 1961).

Following this redistribution occurred as seen by the fall in blood concentration of lignocaine. After an interval a second intravenous infusion was
administered. This gave rise to a precipitous fall in blood pressure associated with an elevation in the blood concentration of the local anaesthetic, and
a convulsion occurred. This was treated immediately by means of a small
dose of barbiturate and methylamphetamine, and there were no untoward
sequelae.

Fig. 28 shows the effect of speed of administration on blood concentration. This is from a series of cases receiving intravenous infusion of
lignocaine and here the speed of the injection has been correlated with the
blood level which has been achieved in each patient. When a given dose of
local anaesthetic is injected slowly, the blood concentration never reaches
very high levels. However, if the same injection is given in a very short space
of time, there is quite a marked elevation in the concentration of circulating

local anaesthetic. Toxic manifestations occur when the membranes of
excitable tissues receive overwhelming concentrations of local anaesthetic,
as outlined by Dr. WOLFE.

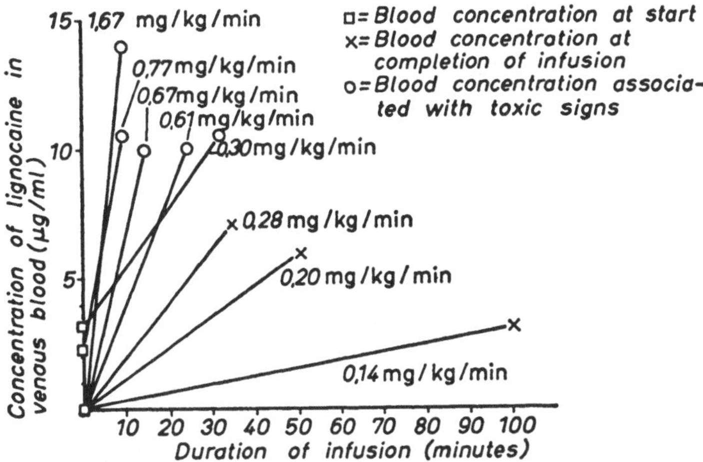

Fig. 28. Blood concentrations of lignocaine at completion of intravenous infusion, related
to dose, rate, and duration of infusion (Bromage and Robson 1961).

I would like to describe a case to show that lignocaine can potentiate
the effects of curare as well as those of succinylcholine (Fig. 29). This was
a chance observation in a patient undergoing a gynaecological operation
during recovery from a dose of 4 mg per stone (0.63 mg/kg) of d-tubocurarine chloride. An infiltration of 100 mg of lignocaine into the perineum
was followed by an increase in the myoneural block of the small muscles of
the hand. The degree of block was monitored by ulnar stimulation with
supramaximal impulses each of 0.1 m sec duration in bursts of 0.3 sec duration and 20 per sec frequency. The ring finger was connected by a linen thread
to a strong flat steel spring myograph recording with ink on a rotating
drum. The perineum had been previously infiltrated with 40 ml of 0.5%
lignocaine and adrenaline 1 : 120,000 shortly after induction of anaesthesia.
This was during the period of maximal depression of the twitch caused by
curare, and thus no effect on the myoneural junction could be observed at
this time. The second injection of only 20 ml of 0.5% lignocaine with
adrenaline 1:120,000 at 90 min after induction of anaesthesia during recovery
from the block can be seen to give rise to a depression of the twitch height.
This effect was transient and did not interfere with the ultimate rate of
recovery following the administration of neostigmine at the end of the
operation. However, it is interesting to note that sufficient absorption of

lignocaine can apparently take place, even in the presence of adrenaline, to cause depression of the neuromuscular junction in the small muscles of the hand.

Colporrhaphy

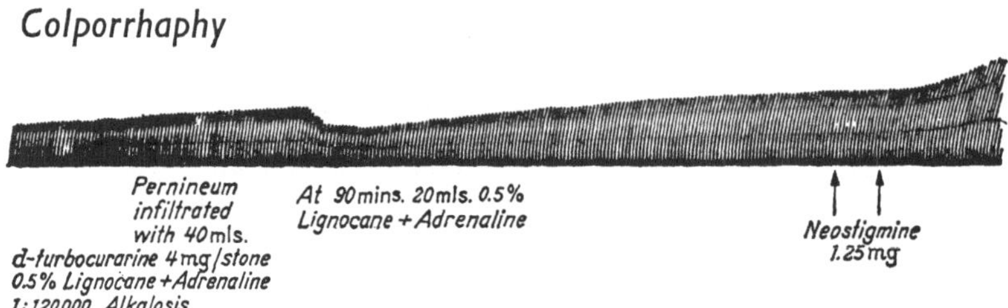

Fig. 29. Summation of d-tubocurarine and lidocaine, with transient depression of finger twitch.

Wolfe: Local anaesthetics injected into the vascular system by accident or design can cause either depression or excitation and convulsions. Which of these effects occurs depends on the blood levels of local anaesthetics in the cerebral circulation and the physiological condition of the patient. High blood levels of local anaesthetics produce convulsions. Dibucaine is one of the most toxic in this regard. Lidocaine on the other hand favours depression and produces sleep patterns in the EEG. Local anaesthetics have been used with some success in the treatment of status epilepticus, particularly in Sweden by Bernhard and Bohm [43].

I would like to mention some of the recent work of Dr. T. C. Baiz at the Montreal Neurological Institute, and I am very grateful to him for allowing me to show two of his figures (30 and 31). Dr. Baiz has studied

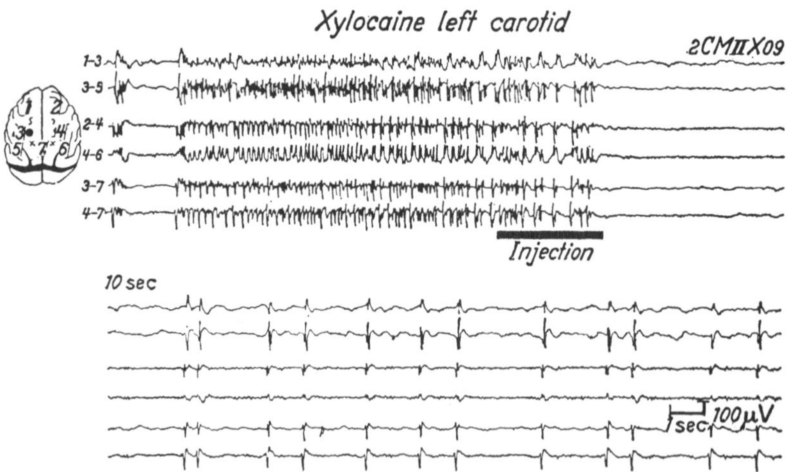

Fig. 30. Electroencephalogram of the monkey with a penicillin focus on the left hemisphere. The figure shows the seizure pattern which was immediately eliminated by injection into the left carotid artery of 0.07 mg/kg Xylocaine.

the effects of xylocaine injected in the carotid artery on seizures induced in monkeys by the application of penicillin to the cortex. Intracarotid xylocaine will cause immediate ipsilateral depression or convulsions, depending on the dosage. However, the therapeutic-toxic range is narrow. Fig. 31 illustrates the development of seizure patterns with ophthalmoplegia, contralateral hemiparesis and clonic movements when 3.3 mg/kg of xylocaine was injected in the left carotid artery. Amytal injection causes synchronization of the EEG. Fig. 30 illustrates the effect of exceedingly small intracarotid injections of xylocaine (0.07 mg/kg) on a penicillin seizure. During the seizure the head and eyes of the monkey were turning to the right with jerking movements of the right forelimb followed by clonic movements in all extremities. Injection of xylocaine stopped the seizure instantly and the animal became alert and immediately ate a banana. This injection afforded protection for 14 min.

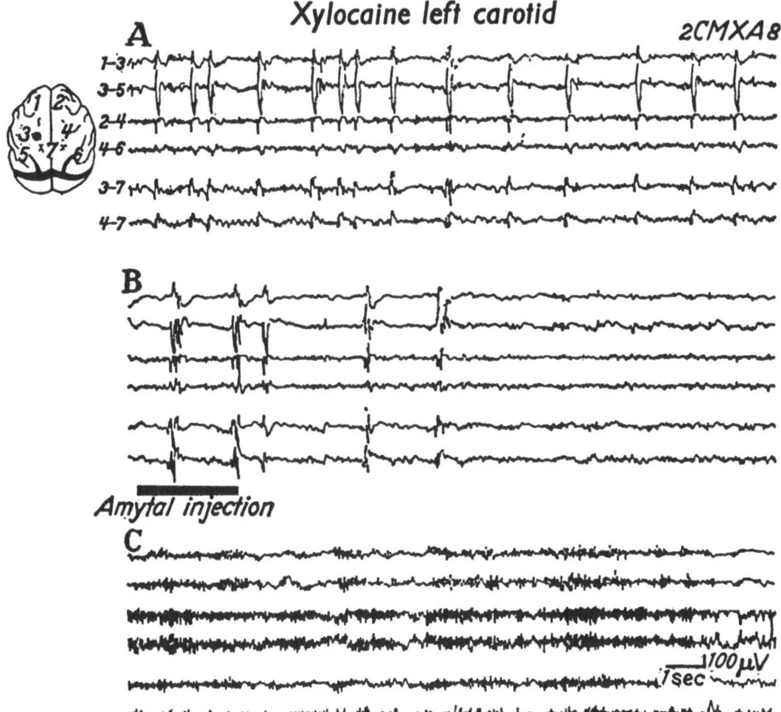

Fig. 31. The effect of Xylocaine on normal cortical activity followed by the effect of sodium amytal on the Xylocaine induced seizure.
3.3 mg/kg xylocaine injected into left carotid artery (10 mg total injected in 0.5 cc). There was no seizure activity from the cortex prior to the injection of Xylocaine. A. 20 seconds after injection of Xylocaine. B. One minute after injection of Xylocaine. 15 mg of sodium amytal was injected into right carotid artery. C. 30 seconds after the injection of sodium amytal. The EEG was normal prior to the injection of Xylocaine.

Chairman: Does the blood concentration of local anaesthetic really mean anything, or should we think in terms of tissue levels, and the time in which equilibrium is established between blood and tissues? For example, if lignocaine is given by rapid intravenous infusion convulsions and cardiovascular depression occur when the blood concentration reaches 10 micrograms per millilitre. And yet we have found that if the drug is absorbed gradually over many hours, blood levels considerably in excess of this threshold may be achieved without convulsions or cardiovascular depression [74].

Eriksson: I am afraid I cannot answer that question completely, but I would like to mention that in experiments carried out by Dr. ENGLESSON, WAHLQVIST, ORTENGREN and myself [75], we found that while we were having blood concentrations that did not change considerably for 30 to 40 min, the volunteers' subjective experiences and objective symptoms that could be seen on EEG, ECG etc., only lasted for about 10 min. This indicates that there might be some difference between the tissue concentrations and the blood concentrations. In other words it is not altogether clear that the blood concentrations always mirror the toxicity.

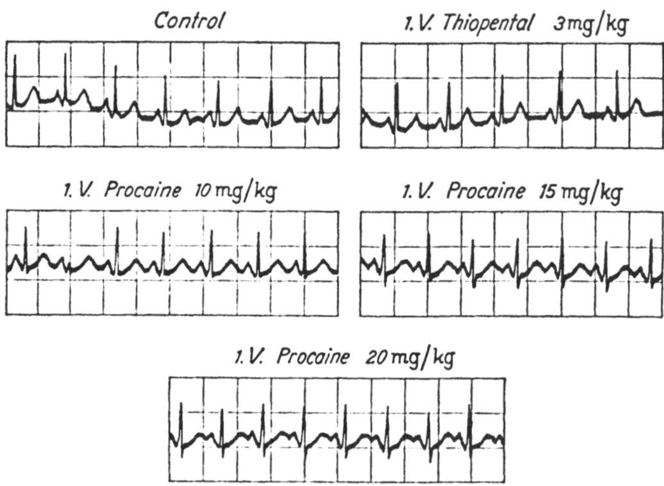

Fig. 32. Intravenous procaine and the ECG.

Usubiaga: I want to comment upon two points Dr. GEDDES has made. The first one is that after inadvertent or deliberate injection of large amounts of local anaesthetic drugs, objective central nervous system effects (convulsions) appear before gross cardiovascular depression. We have found that although the blood pressure may remain normal at the time of convulsions, the electrocardiogram at this time shows not only a sinus tachycardia but a significant depression of the ST segment (Fig. 32). Both of these phenomena revert spontaneously. This cardiac depressant effect is particularly evident after procaine administration.

The second point is closely related and concerns the use of thiopental during the convulsions. The depressant effect of thiopental and local anaesthetics on the cardiovascular system can be additive. But the interaction, we will point out, is not only on the cardiovascular system but also on the central nervous system.

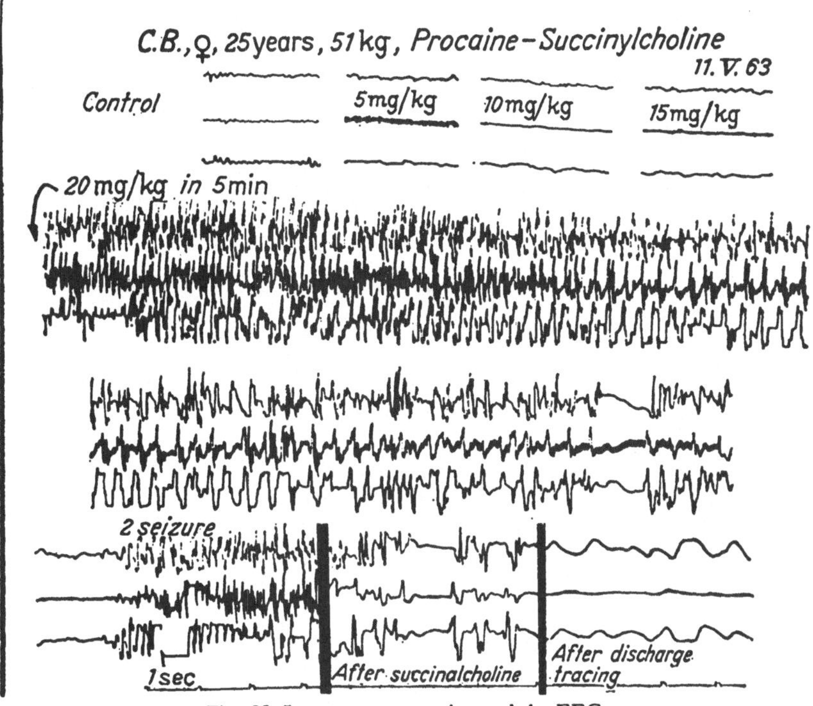

Fig. 33. Intravenous procaine and the EEG.

The intravenous administration of increasing amounts of local anaesthetic drugs in an unpremedicated human volunteer produces on the electroencephalogram a progressive disappearance of the alpha waves, the appeaance of superimposed myograms, and later on, the abrupt onset of the seizure pattern (Fig. 33). This EEG convulsive activity coincides with the initiation of muscle convulsions. Two well defined periods can be described: the first one is composed of high voltage spikes with a frequency of 8 to 12 cycles per second, and these correspond with the generalized tonic muscular contraction. Without any transition the spikes become more separated and rhythmically discharged at a rate corresponding with the clonic muscular phase. Each tonic-clonic burst is separated from the preceding one by a period of electrical inactivity. The mean duration of all convulsive episodes was longer for lidocaine than procaine, lasting up to 3 min in the most prolonged case. Spontaneous ventilation was arrested during the entire period of the convulsion. After the cessation of the electrical seizure a flat after-discharge tracing lasting 10–20 sec was observed, at the end of which, spontaneous ventilation reappeared. Later on, a slow theta rhythm became predominant and in the next 10–15 min there was a gradual return to the preceding alpha rhythm.

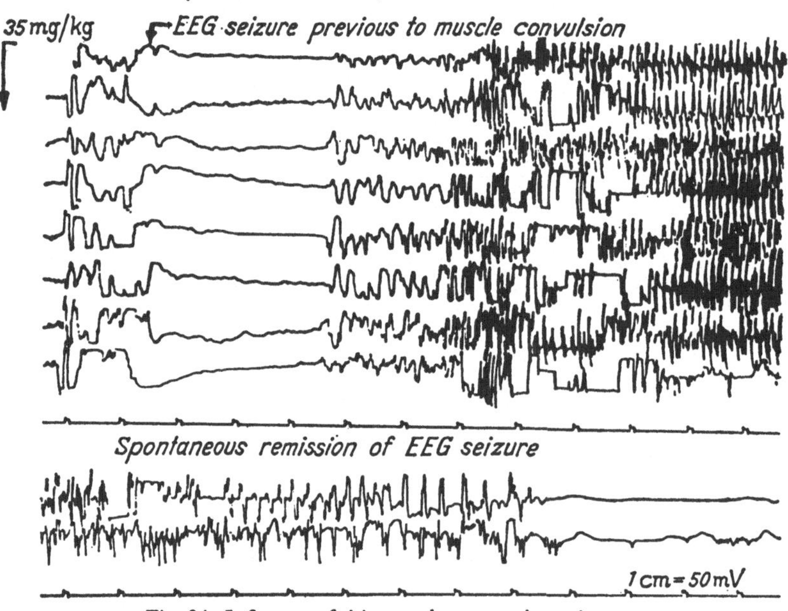

Fig. 34. Influence of thiopental on procaine seizures.

The amount of procaine or lidocaine necessary to develop convulsions was increased when thiopental was injected before the administration of the local anaesthetic drugs. This is illustrated by the case in Fig. 34 where 35 mg/kg of procaine were injected before the appearance of the seizures, in contrast to the 20 mg/kg injected in Fig. 33, in which thiopental was not previously administered. However, thiopental does not prevent the appearance of convulsions, it only delays them. Thiopental injected during the seizures stopped them, shortening mainly the tonic phase. The flat after-discharge pattern observed in the cases of spontaneous remission of the seizures was also modified by intravenous thiopental. Instead of the flat local anaesthetic-like pattern, the fast microwaves of thiopental appeared as shown in Fig. 35.

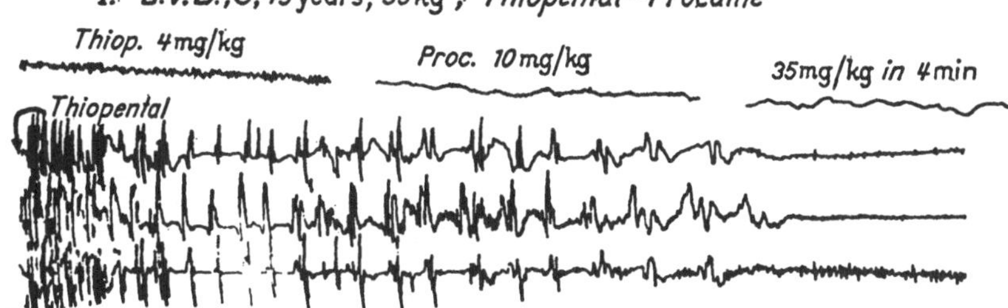

Fig. 35. Effect of thiopental on established procaine seizures.

Succinylcholine has been reported by ACHESON [76] to increase the convulsive activity of lidocaine in cats, but we have not been able to confirm this, nor on the neurotoxicity of lidocaine following the previous administration of succinylcholine. There was neither increase in the length of convulsions nor changes in the EEG pattern with successive injections using the same subject as his own control.

The different patterns observed after the spontaneous cessation of the local anaesthetic convulsions, compared with the cessation after the injection of thiopental, suggest that the place of action of the two drugs is different. Thiopental acts preferentially on the Ascending Reticular System. In the case of local anaesthetics there is increasing evidence showing that an inhibition of the subcortical amygdalar system takes place [77, 78].

We believe that the anticonvulsive, analgesic and the later convulsant actions of local anaesthetics are due to an increasing and progressive depression of the central nervous system.

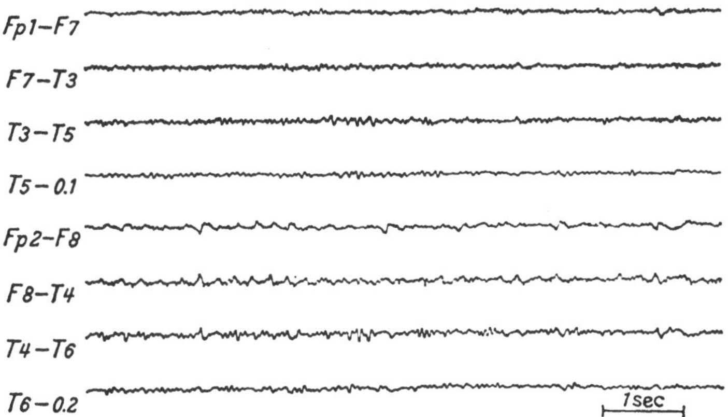

Fig. 36. EEG before injection of 15 mls of 1 % Xylocaine showing a marked sharp wave activity in the right fronto-temporal region. The position of the electrodes according to the 10–20 system.

Eriksson: It is well known that large doses of anaesthetics give rise to convulsions. It was therefore quite a surprise when Swedish researchers, about ten years ago, published reports that some of these local anaesthetics were able to help in epileptic convulsions. A dentist, Halldin [79] was the first to publish this. Bernhard and Bohm [80] however, have written a number of papers on this subject, and have clearly demonstrated that Xylocaine and also some other local anaesthetics can stop epileptic convulsions for some time. Fig. 36 shows an EEG from a patient with a continuous focal epilepsy. This is taken from an unpublished investigation by Dr. A Persson and myself, done at the Department of Neurophysiology at the Karolinska Hospital in Stockholm. The EEG shows continuous focal sharp waves, and the patient had continuous clonic convulsions in his left leg. After injection of 150 mg of Xylocaine intravenously, the EEG turned almost normal and the epileptic fits stopped (Fig. 37). He had no convulsions for about 10–11 min, then the fits and the pathological EEG returned. The dose of Xylocaine required for blocking these epileptic convulsions is somewhat lower than the one needed to provoke convulsions. You generally do not need more than 100 mg in a single dose to be able to stop an epileptic convulsion.

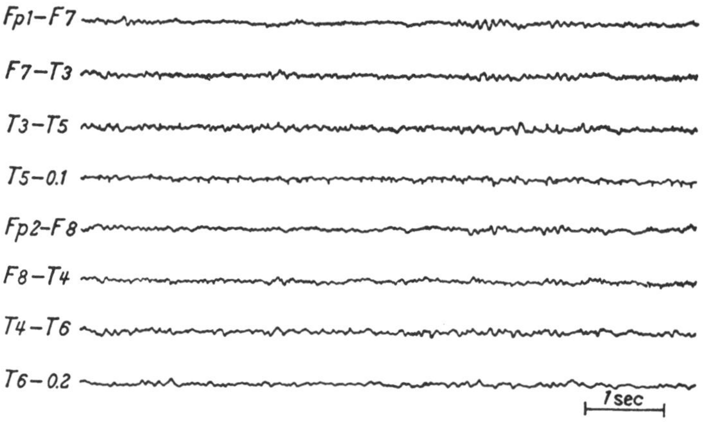

Fig. 37. EEG two minutes after Xylocaine. No epileptogenic activity visible.

Geddes: Maykut and Kalow [81] showed that there is some degree of summation between the toxic effects of the local anaesthetics and the depressant actions of barbiturates. Clinically this is very important. If you are treating convulsions with a barbiturate, the dose should be kept as low as possible, otherwise you may get a summation of central toxic actions as Dr. Usubiaga has pointed out.

Chairman: I would like the panel to discuss the influence of the blood gases and the ionic environment on the toxicity of local anaesthetics. Asphyxia and local anaesthetic toxicity have many points in common. Moreover, the changes in hydrogen ion concentration associated with respiratory acidosis affect the degree of ionization of circulating local anaesthetic drugs and their disposition within the body.

The basic components of asphyxia, hypoxaemia and hypercarbia, are depressant to smooth muscle, and summate with local anaesthetics to exacerbate the cardiovascular depression. In Fig. 27 shown by Dr. GEDDES, it can be seen that during an overdose of intravenous lidocaine a convulsion was preceded by hypoventilation and arterial hypotension. In this situation one suspects that a vicious circle develops in the following manner: Depression → asphyxia → cellular acidosis → increased cellular uptake of local anaesthetic → more depression. I would suggest that a vicious circle mechanism of this sort is at the core of these toxic reactions and that clinically it can be prevented, or possibly broken, by hyperventilation and respiratory alkalosis.

In parts of South America where nitrous oxide has been in scarce supply, very large doses of local anaesthetics are commonly used to produce generalized analgesia and unconsciousness, and a total dose of 3 or 4 or more grams of procaine is quite usual during an abdominal operation, and yet cardiovascular depression is very rare. Now these patients are all hyperventilated with 100 per cent oxygen, and it would seem that the high oxygen tension and the respiratory alkalosis are at least partially protective.

Eriksson: GRANBERG and I came across this problem in a rather unexpected way, when we studied the renal clearances for Xylocaine and Citanest [82]. We were trying to see whether by increasing the osmotic diuresis we could also increase the amount of local anaesthetic that was being excreted. So, to some of the volunteers that got Xylocaine in the mixture of inulin, PAH and a local anaesthetic, we gave a rather rapid infusion of 500 millilitres of 20 per cent mannitol at the end of the experiment, in order to increase the diuresis. We were quite surprised by the result. The subjects had had some minor toxic symptoms when they received the priming dose of 100 mg of Xylocaine, with corresponding amounts of inulin and PAH. These symptoms were from the central nervous system and consisted of sleepiness, sensation of cold, auditory disturbances etc. When we gave the mannitol these toxic symptoms returned and in some of the cases they were more severe than during the priming dose. The mannitol diuresis however, did not raise the clearance for Xylocaine. Fig. 38 shows the three experiments we did with Xylocaine and mannitol. When we started giving mannitol we produced a dilution of the plasma, and the hematocrit fell. The plasma concentrations of Xylocaine in two of the subjects first fell somewhat, but then went up and rose to values even higher than earlier. One subject experienced such alarming toxic symptoms that we had to stop the mannitol infusion. Even after we had stopped it the toxic symptoms continued for a while. It is a little difficult to interpret this from a clinical point of view. It could be that we withdrew so much water from the cells that there would be proportionally more local anaesthetic left. The resulting dehydration might also give rise to an intracellular acidosis, so it is possible that once again changes of pH may explain the findings.

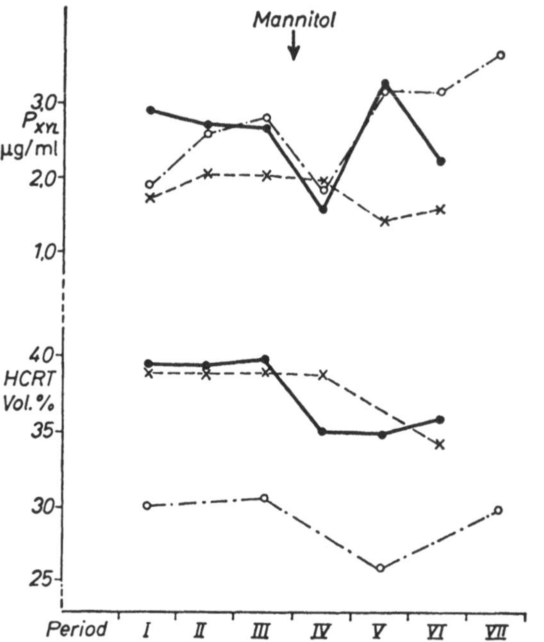

Fig. 38. Effect of mannitol on the plasma concentration of Xylocaine and the hematocrit. 500 ml of 20 % mannitol were given intravenously during 15–20 minutes. The mannitol gave a dilution of the plasma with a lowering of the plasma level of Xylocaine and the hematocrit. In spite of a low and constant hematocrit the plasma level of Xylocaine increased in two of the cases and reached values higher than earlier in the experiment.

Chairman: Finally we must come to the question of toxicity from breakdown products of the local anaesthetics. When large amounts of local anaesthetic such as procaine are administered intravenously it is common to see a peripheral cyanosis of the lips and finger nails, despite high inspired oxygen tensions. A blood sample drawn from these patients does not become pink when shaken with oxygen, and the dark colouration is due to methaemoglobin.

Methaemoglobin formation can be caused by many aniline and phenol derivatives, such as are formed from the breakdown of local anaesthetics. These interfere with the oxidation-reduction enzymes of the red cell, allowing the ferrous iron of haemoglobin to become oxidized to the ferric state.

This oxidation process is reversible with methylene blue, up to a point, but if carried too far leads to Heinz-body formation and death of the red-cell [83].

Eriksson: It is known that some different local anaesthetics produce methaemoglobinaemia. Procaine is one, Benzocaine another, and Citanest has recently been shown to do so too. Citanest, as you know, has a very low toxicity which allows the use of large amounts in single doses. In Japan, Sweden, the U. K. and the U. S., investigators when using high doses – over one gram – found that the patients developed cyanosis some hours later. This is explained by the fact that Citanest gives rise to methaemoglobinaemia. D'Amato [84] among others has studied this problem and showed that the methaemoglobinaemia can be reversed by methylene blue. HOLM-DAHL and HJELM in Uppsala, Sweden [85] have shown that with doses of Citanest around 600 mg, the degree of methaemoglobinaemia will be 4–6 per cent of the total haemoglobin concentration, and this is a fairly low value from the clinical point of view. At the symposium on Citanest in Santos, September 1964[1] this problem was thoroughly discussed and it was generally agreed that this degree of methaemoglobinaemia is of little clinical significance. In the cases that had a more pronounced cyanosis and higher values of methaemoglobinaemia, rather large doses of Citanest, sometimes 4–5 times the amount usually needed for a surgical block were used.

Chairman: Thank you gentlemen, our time is up.

References

[1] GEDDES, I. C. and J. H. QUASTEL: Anesthesiology **17**, 666 (1956).
[2] KINI, M. M. and J. H. QUASTEL: Science **131**, 412 (1960).
[3] ANDERSON, N. B. and J. S. GRAVENSTEIN: J. Pharmacol., **147**, 40 (1965).
[4] ANDERSON, N. B.: Anesth. Analg. **43**, 49 (1964).
[5] QUASTEL, J. H.: In Neurochemistry ed. Elliott, K.A.C., Page, I.H. and Quastel, J. H. Charles C. Thomas, Springfield, Illinois 790 (1962).
[6] LARRABEE, M. G. and J. D. KLINGMAN: In Neurochemistry ed. Elliott, K.A.C., Page, I.H. and Quastel, J. H. Charles C. Thomas, Springfield, Illinois 172 (1962).
[7] GREIG, M. E. and A. J. GIBBON: Science **123**, 939 (1956).
[8] SHANES, A. H.: Pharmacol. Rev., **10**, 59 (1958).
[9] KAVENAU, J. LEE: Structure and function in biological membranes. Vol. 1. Holden-Day Inc., San Francisco, 1965.
[10] DAVSON, H. A. and J. F. DANIELLI: The permeability of natural membranes. Cambridge Univ. Press, 1943.
[11] ROBERTSON, J. D.: Progress in Biophysics, **10**, 343 (1960).

---

[1] Symposium on Citanest, Acta anesthesiologica Scandanavica. Supplement XVI, 1965.

[12] STOECKENIUS, W.: The interpretation of Ultrastructure, R. J. C. HARRIS, ed., Academic Press, N. Y., p. 349; Circulation 26, 1066 (1962).

[13] FERNANDEZ-MORAN, H.: Circulation 26, 1039 (1962); J. Cell Biol., 22, 63 (1964); J. Roy. Micros. Soc., 83, 183 (1964).

[14] FERNANDEZ-MORAN, H.: In Ultrastructure and Metabolism of the Nervous System, Vol. 40, A.R.N.M.D. Research Publ. p. 235 (1962).

[15] WATSON, P. J.: J. Pharm. Pharmacol., 12, 257 (1960).

[16] TOMAN, J. E. P.: in Neurochemistry ed. etc. p. 728 (1962).

[17] CONDOURIS, G. A.: J. Pharmacol. 131, 243 (1961); 141, 253 (1963).

[18] BENNETT, A. L. and K. G. CHINBURG: J. Pharmacol. 88, 72 (1946).

[19] THESLEFF, S.: Acta Physiol. Scand., 37, 335 (1956).

[20] EHRENPREIS, S.: Biochim. Biophys. Acta, 44, 561 (1960); in Bioelectrogenesis, ed. C. Chargas and A. Paes de Carvalho, Elsevier, Amsterdam, p. 379, 1961.

[21] TOBIAS, J. M., D. P. AGIN, and R. PAWLOWSKI: J. Gen. Physiol., 45, 989 (1962).

[22] ACEVES, J. and X. MACHNE: J. Pharmacol., 140, 38 (1963).

[23] TASAKI, I.: in Neurophysiology Vol. 75, Amer. Physiol. Soc. Publ., 1959; J. Gen. Physiol., 46, 755 (1963); Proc. Natn. Acad. Sc., 48, 1177 (1962); 50, 619 (1963); 52, 804 (1964).

[24] LING, G. N.: A physical theory of the living state. Blaisdell Publ. Co., New York, 1962.

[25] WEBER, A.: J. Biol. Chem., 234 (1959); J. Gen. Physiol., 46, 679 (1963).

[26] HUXLEY, A. F. and R. W. STRAUB: J. Physiol., 143, 40 (1958).

[29] HUXLEY, H. F.: Nature, 202, 1067 (1964).

[30] EBASHI, S. and F. LIPMAN: J. Cell Biol., 14, 389 (1962).

[31] HASSELBACH, W. and M. MAKINOSE: Biochem. Biophys. Res. Comm., 7, 132 (1962).

[32] KUPERMAN, A. S., OKAMOTO, M., BEYER, A. M. and W. A. VOLPERT: Science, 144, 1222 (1964).

[33] SKOU, J. C.: Acta Pharmacol. Toxicol., 10, 235 (1954).

[34] CLEMENTS, J. A. and K. M. WILSON: Proc. Natl. Acad. Sc., 48, 1008 (1962).

[35] GADDUM, J. H.: Pharmacology, 5th Edn., Oxford Univ. Press, p. 178, 1959.

[36] TRUANT, A. P. and B. TAKMAN: Anesth. Analg., 38, 478 (1959).

[37] ADRIANI, J.: Clin. Pharmacol. Ther., 1, 645 (1960).

[38] WEATHERBY, J. H. and H. B. HAAG: in Pharmacology in Medicine, ed. V. A. Drill, McGraw-Hill, London, p. 99 1958.

[39] TREVAN, J. W. and E. BOOCK: Brit. J. Exptl. Path. 8, 478 (1959).

[40] RITCHIE, J. M. and P. GREENGARD: J. Pharmacol. 133, 241 (1961).

[41] LORENTE DE NO, R.: J. Cell. Comp. Physiol., 35, 195, 203 (1950)., J. Gen. Physiol., 35, 203 (1951).

[42] LORENTE DE NO, R. and G. A. CONDOURIS: Proc. Natl. Acad. Sc., 45, 592 (1959).

[43] BERNHARD, C. G. and E. BOHM: Experientia, 10, 474 (1954); Brit. J. Pharmacol., 10, 288 (1955).

[44] BROWN, G. L. and J. S. GILLESPIE: J. Physiol., 138, 81 (1957).

[45] WHITBY, L. G., G. HERTHING and J. AXELROD: Nature 187, 604 (1960); J. Pharmacol., 134, 146 (1961).

[46] FURCHGOTT, R. F., S. M. KIRPEKAR, M. RICHER and A. SCHWARB: J. Pharmacol., 142, 39 (1963).

[47] KIRPEKAR, S. M. and P. CERVONI: J. Pharmacol., 142, 59 (1963).

[48] GRAHAM, N. H., F. M. ABBOUD and J. W. ECKSTEIN: J. Pharmacol., 143, 340 (1964).

[49] KIRPEKAR, S. M., P. CERVONI and D. COURI: J. Pharmacol. 142, 71 (1963).

[50] BLASCHKO, H., G. V. R. BORN, A. D'IORIO and M. R. EADE: J. Physiol., 133, 548 (1956).
[51] SCHUMANN, H. J.: Arch. Exptl. Path. Pharmacol. 233, 237 (1958).
[52] BIANCHI, C.: Farmaco, Ediz. Sci. 10, 78 (1955).
[53] WIEDLING, S.: Xylocaine, Almqvist and Wiksell, Stockholm, 1964.
[54] HIGMAN, H. B. and E. BARTELS: Biochim. biophys. Acta, 44, 561 (1961).
[55] LOWENSTEIN, W. R.: Ann. New York Acad. Sci. Current problems in electro-biology (D. P. Purpura, Ed.) 94, 337, 1961.
[56] FOLDES, F., DAVIS, D. L. and O. J. PLEKSS: Anesthesiol. 17, 187, 1956.
[57] MIESCHER, K.: Helv. Chim. Acta. 15, 163, 1932.
[58] LOFGREN, N.: Xylocaine. Haeggstroms, Stockholm, 1948.
[59] BULLOCK, K., and J. GRUNDY: J. Pharm. and Pharmacol. 7, 755, 1955.
[60] LOOMIS, W. F.: Science, 126, 735, 1957.
[61] CALDWELL, P. C.: J. Physiol (Lond) 142, 22, 1958.
[62] HALPERN, B. N. and R. BINAGHI: Nature 183, 1397, 1959.
[63] BROMAGE, P. R.: Citanest: Acta anaesthetica Scand. Suppl. XVI, 55, 1965.
[64] ERIKSSON, E.: Acta anaesthetica Scand. 5, 191, 1961.
[65] BROMAGE, P. R.: Brit. med. J. 2, 1634, 1962.
[66] BROMAGE, P. R.: Canad. med. Assoc. J. 85, 1136, 1961.
[67] GEDDES, I. C.: Anesthesie Analgesie Reanimation. 15, 908, 1958.
[68] SUNG, C. Y. and A. P. TRUANT: J. Pharmacol. exper. Ther. 113, 433, 1954.
[69] HOLLUNGER, G.: Acta pharmacol. (Kbh). 17, 365, 1960.
[70] GEDDES, I. C.: Citanest: Acta anaesthetica Scand. Suppl. XVI, 21, 1965.
[71] ERIKSSON, E. and P. O. GRANBERG: Citanest: Acta anaesthetica Scand. Suppl. XVI, 59, 1965.
[72] MILNE, M. D., B. H. SCRIBNER and M. A. CRAWFORD: Amer. J. Med. 24, 709, 1958.
[73] KALOW, W. J.: Pharmacol. exper. Ther. 104, 1221, 1952.
[74] BROMAGE, P. R. and J. G. ROBSON: Anaesthesia 16, 461, 1961.
[75] ENGLESSON, S., E. ERIKSSON, S. WAHLQUIST and B. ORTENGREN: First European Congress of Anesthesiology Proceedings 2, 206, 1962.
[76] ACHESON, F., A. B. BULL and P. GLEES: Anaesthesiology 17, 802, 1956.
[77] ERDELBERG, E., H. LESSE and F. GAULT: First International Pharmacology Meeting, 214, Pergamon Press Book, New York, 1963.
[78] DE JONG, R. H. and I. H. WAGMANN: Fed. Proc. 22, 187, 1963.
[79] HALLDIN, T.: Svenska Läkartidn. Vol. 51, 2147, 1954.
[80] BERNHARD, C. G. and E. BOHM: Acta Physiol. Scand. 31, Suppl. 114, 5, 1954.
[81] MAYKUT, M. O. and W. KALOW: Canad. Anaesth. Soc. J. 2, 109, 1955.
[82] ERIKSSON, E. and P. O. GRANBERG: Citanest: Acta Anaesth. Scand. Suppl. XVI, 1965.
[83] DE LEEUW, N. K., L. SHAPIRO and L. LOWENSTEIN: Ann. Int. Med. 58, 592, 1963.
[84] D'AMATO, H. E.: To be published.
[85] HJELM, M. and M. H. HOLMDAHL: Citanest: Acta Anaesth. Scand. Suppl. XVI, 1965.

E. Necessity and functions of an autonomous department of anaesthesiology

Chairman: J. A. Nesi, Caracas
Members: L. Bianchetti (in absence of E. Ciocatto), Turin; K. Iwatsuki, Sendai; L. de Freitas Brandao, Porto Alegre; H. Poulsen, Aarhus.

Nesi: Señores, damos comienzo a la discusión del tema «La Necesidad y las Funciones de un Departamento Autónomo de Anestesiología». Yo creo que el objeto de este Panel no es explicar lo bueno que es un departamento de Anestesiología, ni lo felices que somos algunos de nosotros por tener un departamento de Anestesiología bien constituído; sino más bien, cuáles son las dificultades y las limitaciones que pueden encontrarse en distintos países y en distintas condiciones, para organizar un departamento de Anestesiología, y cuáles son las condiciones básicas para su funcionamiento. Para conseguir este objetivo, hemos reunido en la Mesa a representantes de países de distintas latitudes del mundo, pero tratando de elegir aquéllos que presentaran cierta similitud, tanto en densidad de población y condiciones socio-económicas, como en evolución histórica de la Anestesiología.

Como no soy yo el que va a tratar el tema, sino los Miembros de la Mesa y los del público, a quienes ya invito formalmente a intervenir en la discusión, voy a comenzar el programa pidiendo a cada uno de los participantes que expongan su opinión y su experiencia personal sobre cuatro puntos fundamentales que, para mayor claridad, he pedido que se proyecten en la pantalla.

El Prof. Ciocatto es uno de los Miembros del Panel, pero desgraciadamente debe participar en este momento en otra reunión, de modo que, momentáneamente, va a tomar su lugar su Primer Asistente, el Dr. Bianchetti, a quién le ruego que nos explique brevemente su experiencia en Torino.

Bianchetti: Je m'exuse si la pauvre connaissance du français ne me permet pas de m'expliquer suffisamment. Je chercherai de vous donner, en deux mots, une description de l'anesthésie en Italie, et surtout à Turin, où nous travaillons. Il y a à peu près quinze ans que l'anesthésie en Italie a pris son aspect scientifique et officiel. En effet, on a commencé l'Ecole de

Spécialisation en 1950. Aujourd'hui il y a à peu près 500 anesthésistes, qui se sont spécialisés aux Ecoles de Spécialisation que presque chaque Université possède. En Italie, aujourd'hui, presque toutes les anesthésies sont faites exclusivement par des médecins spécialisés. La loi italienne permet que chaque médecin, qui a le diplôme de médecin-chirugien, peut pratiquer toute thérapeutique, toutes les méthodes, et donner même des anesthésies.

En ce qui concerne l'organisation des services d'anesthésiologie, en Italie, on peut dire aujourd'hui, que presque tous les hôpitaux ont envisagé ou ont réalisé des services d'anesthésiologie; mais cette situation-là on la voit seulement dans les grands hôpitaux et dans les hôpitaux des grandes villes, tandis que plusieurs hôpitaux de centres plus petits ne comptent pas encore avec un service indépendant, et les anesthésies sont faites par des anesthésistes ou bien par des médecins avec quelque pratique d'anesthésie, mais qui ne sont pas des professionnels spécialisés. Au côté des méthodes standard d'anesthésie employées couramment, les techniques plus évolues, comme hypotension controlée, hypothermie, neuroléptoanalgésie, sont employées en plusieurs hôpitaux avec une connaissance suffisante des problèmes qui sont posés par ces types d'anesthésie.

En ce qui concerne le titre de spécialisation en anesthésie, on peut l'obtenir dans presque toutes les Universités italiennes, après une période de deux années d'études et des examens qu'ont lieu à la fin de chaque année ou bien à la fin du cours; ceci peut-être une thèse ou discussion sur un sujet choisi, pour permettre à l'anesthésiste de démontrer sa préparation théorique et pratique. Nous souhaitons que cette période de spécialisation pourra être amenée bientôt à trois années.

Quant au programme pour l'avenir nous pensons que pour atteindre l'optimum de nos aspirations il faut commencer pour constituer des services d'anesthésie centralisés et complètement autonomes. Jusqu'au présent cette condition n'a pu s'étendre à tous les hôpitaux italiens, et il y a encore beaucoup d'anesthésistes qui travaillent seulement pour un département de chirurgie ou seulement pour un chirurgien. Nous souhaitons que cette situation lá pourra changer dans les prochaines années. Mais ce que à notre avis est plus important pour la réalisation de notre programme c'est, à part la centralisation des services, la possibilité de leur confier un rôle complètement autonome pour la réanimation, sous tous les points de vue, et surtout pour la thérapeutique de la douleur. C'est le développement de ces activités parallèles aux services rendus ordinairement aux chirurgiens qui nous permettra obtenir plus facilement une vraie autonomie.

Nesi: Muchas gracias, Dr. BIANCHETTI. Ahora voy a pedir al Dr. KENICHI IWATSUKI que, siguiendo el mismo orden, nos refiera la experiencia en Japón.

Iwatsuki: Before discussing the subjects in detail, I would like to refer briefly to the present status of anaesthesia in Japan, and also present some of the problems that our profession is confronted with. In Japan, it can be said that modern anaesthesia started after the war – actually in 1950. In 1950 Dr. MEYER SAKLAD visited Japan as a member of the Unitarian Service Committee and greatly contributed to open the mind of leading Japanese surgeons to the true meaning of anaesthesia and also to stimulate interest in anaesthesiology among young doctors.

In 1952, a Department of Anaesthesiology was established in Tokyo University for the first time, and Dr. YAMAMURA was assigned as the Professor of Anaesthesiology. Since then, other medical schools have followed, and now, among 46 medical schools, there are 18 schools with Professor of Anaesthesiology, and 18 others with Assistant Professor or Instructor, heading the Departments. In each of them a number of doctors are taking training. In 1954, the Japan Society of Anaesthesiology was established. But, as you can imagine from this name, it is not composed exclusively of specialists in anaesthesia, but embraces all doctors who are interested in the science of anaesthesia. The members are now approximately 1500, which do not necessarily represent the specialists in anaesthesia. At present one of the problems we are confronted with is the shortage of specialists in anaesthesia. This may be a trend not only in Japan, as reported in the morning session. It is true that there exist various reasons, some of them are specially limited to Japan, but some others may be inherent in this speciality. Here I would like to give you a brief account of the professional status of the doctors engaged in anaesthesia in Japan. In our country, until four years ago, anaesthesia was not included in the list of medical branches officially approved by the law. We had long felt the need for ammending the law, and in 1960 we succeeded in making a new system of certifying doctors engaged in the practice of anaesthesia. Under this system, an applicant having specified qualification, who satisfied the screening board, is given a certification by the Minister of Public Welfare. This . . . The privilege of this certification is that the doctors can profess or advertise anaesthesia officially as his field of medical practice. This is difficult to translate into English, but it may be said "certification junior grade". The following are the qualifications. Number I: any medical doctors who have experienced anaesthesia of more than 300 cases, using gas machines, over the period of two years. Number II: any medical doctors who have undergone training of anaesthesia for more than two years at the approved departments of anaesthesia, not only in Japan but also in foreign countries. By the end of August this year, 958 doctors have certified in this manner. However, not all of the doctors certified in this manner are specialists in anaesthesia. Actually quite a number of them are surgeons and giving anaesthesia in part-time. The full-time anaesthesiologists are approximately $^1/_5$ of them.

This certification seemed unsatisfactory for the full-time specialist. Therefore in 1962, we started another system. This can be said "certification senior grade", which requests for the applicant more strict qualifications than the previous junior grade. The applicant should have a career of at least five year full-time practice, including two years of special training. Certification is given to them, when they pass the written, oral and practical examinations conducted by the Board of the Japan Society of Anaesthesiology. There are 64 doctors who are certified in this system until now. They are taking a most active part as a chief, or leading staffs, or instructors in the anaesthesia departments in the universities or in other big hospitals. This is one more step to pave the way toward specialization. The other point I would like to refer to is the economic problem. So far as our country is concerned, doctors engaged in anaesthesia, are working in hospitals on salary basis without the privilege of having private cases, and at the same time it is difficult for them to do private practice on private fee basis because of the health insurance system. Under this system, the medical fee is fixed by the law. This seems to be one of the reasons why the doctors who enter this speciality are still small in number. In order to cover the shortage of specialists in anaesthesiology, there has been a move to allow nurses to administer anaesthesia. However we have kept a firm stand against such a move. Now we have no nurse anaesthetists. Recently, the activities of anaesthesiologists are becoming widened outside the operating theater, as you have already known. They are taking care not only of the post-operative patients, but also of the non-surgical patients with respiratory or cardiovascular insufficiencies, as well as those suffering from intractable pains. Pain clinic was established for the first time in August 1962 in Tokyo University Hospital, which was followed by other university hospitals recently. Nerve blocks, occasionally sympathetic ganglion blocks, are the principal procedures, and the results are very satisfactory and encouraging. As the last subject, I would like to refer briefly to the teaching of anaesthesiology in the university hospitals in Japan. Anaesthesiology itself is not yet included in the obligatory subjects of medical education, but a lecture of anaesthesiology, including oxygen therapy and resuscitation, has been given to medical students in the majority of medical schools. So far as our medical school is concerned, we have 36 hours for basic science of anaesthesiology and 24 hours of practical training in the third and fourth year. Internes are arranged to rotate in the anaesthesia department for two weeks. It is almost similar in all medical schools. In 15 universities there is a post-graduate course of 4 years and the students are given a diploma of PhD, when they present the dissertation and pass the final examination. In regard to the post-graduate education, as I mentioned previously, doctors who are going to be qualified as specialists or instructors in anaesthesia, are requested to take a special training at the Department of Anaesthesiology for at least two years, followed by full-

time practice of anaesthesia for more than three years. Autonomy of an
Anaesthesia Department is without doubt an ideal to be sought. But there
are still many problems before us. I do hope that this Panel will pave the
way to approach the ideal and bring about some solution to the problems
which we are confronted with at present.

Nesi: Muchas gracias, Dr. Iwatsuki. El Dr. Lafayette de Freitas
Brandao expondrá ahora sus puntos de vista en relación con el estado actual
en Brasil.

de Freitas Brandao: Os problemas de anestesia nos hospitais do Brasil
estão em função de cinco variáveis principais: cirurgião, paciente, organização hospitalar, anestesista e sistema de atendimento. A falta de ensino
organizado da anestesia em todo o território nacional, impiediou o entrosamento oficial e lógico entre a anestesia e as cátedras de cirurgia, fazendo
com que ainda um grande número de cirurgiões tolere a anestesia como uma
necessidade, mas não a aceita como parte integrante e inerente ao ato
cirúrgico ou a qualquer procedimento diagnóstico. Em função do sistema
de atendimento, a fixação e a dependencia do paciente ao cirurgião, com
quem inicia seu contato médico, fazem com que seja superestimado o ato
cirúrgico de forma isolada, tornando-o incapaz de raciocinar de forma global
e valorizar convenientemente aspectos isolados de um mesmo conjunto.
As organizações hospitalares foram estruturadas com objectivos diversos: inicialmente com finalidades religiosas e caritativas; posteriormente
com objetivos comerciais e lucrativos puros e, em etapa mais avançada,
com finalidades assistenciais e de ensino, devendo ser constatado de uma
forma genérica, ser diverso e variado o número de organizações que imprópriamente se denominam «hospitais» e «Casas de Saúde». Não ser efetivamente aceita a idea de que «hospital» é organismo técnico, dinámico, de
obrigação e com obrigações comunitárias. Haver uma falta de orientação
médico-técnica efetiva nas Direções e Administrações hospitalares, por
omissão, comodismo e inexperiencia do médico. Haver tolerancia ou omissão
de órgãos e organizações oficias, responsáveis pela melhoria de padrões
técnico-hospitalares e condições de segurança ao paciente, tais como o
Ministério da Saúde e Associações Médicas. Haver do ponto de vista jurídico,
prácticamente ausencia de responsabilidade médico-legal. Haver uma permanente aceitação por parte do médico, de todos êsses problemas e situações. Finalmente, como uma resultante de todos êsses fatores, situa-se o
anestesista, aceitando condições e locais de trabalho desconfortáveis, deficitários e, grande número de vezes, condenáveis e inseguros. En muitas
circunstancias, ainda competindo com a própria organização hospitalar, a
qual encara a realização de anestesias como um procedimento técnico de
execução simples, e como fonte de renda pura. Aceitando, sem que disso se
aperceba, parte da responsabilidade, e sendo conivente com a falta de con-

dições de segurança ao paciente, representada básicamente por falta de condições de recuperação pósanestésica, seja por falta de enfermagem capaz, seja por falta de equipamento técnico, ou pela combinação de ambos.

O sistema de atendimento mais corrente pode ser agrupado em tres formas principais: atendimento isolado, prestado a entidades assistenciais, de ensino, ou a um grupo reduzido de cirurgiões; atendimento em grupo, com finalidades técnicas, económicas, ou com ambas; e finalmente, através de serviços ou Departamentos de Anestesia. Como fatos de interesse em relação ao presente tópico, deve ser ressaltado: a) que a forma predominante é a formação de grupos de anestesistas com finalidades técnicas e económicas; b) que é elevado o número de anestesistas que fazem a especialidade em tempo integral; c) que existem Estados da União nos quais os anestesistas nao aceitam empregos, trabalhando apenas por tarefa; d) que, do ponto de vista económico, o maior interesse de atendimento recai nos Institutos de Previdência Social.

Como opinião pessoal e crítica aos sistemas em uso no Brasil, diríamos o seguinte: dentro das organizações médicas brasileiras, no sentido classista, a Sociedade de Anestesia é a única organizada e estruturada em todo o território nacional, devendo-se isso a um trabalho continuado e eficiente da Sociedade Brasileira de Anestesiologia, desde o início de sua fundção. Do ponto de vista financeiro, em função da remuneração por tarefa, o sistema permite uma remuneração elevada. Permite a livre escôlha, por parte do cirugião, a quem é delegado o direito de escôlher o anestesista que deverá atende-lo. Do ponto de vista médicotécnico, impede a uniformidade de técnica e padronização de condutas, tornando o atendimento incômodo e difícil pela diversidade de locais de trabalho, exigencias de material e equipamento em diversos hospitais, e contrariando, a nosso ver, uma condição inerente a um serviço ou departamento de anestesia que deve ser centralizado em um único local. Com relação á experiencia pessoal, soluções encontradas, etc., pensamos o seguinte: parece-nos difícil pretender, no cenário geográfico brasileiro, estabelecer soluções padronizadas para todos os problemas. Entendemos que como objetivo comum, em cada região deve haver uma adaptação das situações as condições humanas, economicas, sociais e intelectuais existentes, que são diversas.

Os comentários que fazemos representam a experiencia pessoal no extremo Sul do Brasil e resultam da observação e conhecimento dos problemas da classe médica em nosso Estado, das organizações hospitalares, dos problemas de enfermagem, da legislação e estruturação do ensino universitário, por atuação direta e indireta nesses setores durante vários anos. Pretendemos, em função disso, atingir os objetivos desejados, dirigindo o nosso esforço nos seguintes pontos: 1) trabalho de esclarecimento e doutrinação junto as cúpulas universitárias es associações médicas; 2) trabalho de esclarecimento informativo e formativo junto ao estudante ed

medicina, no sentido de mostrar-lhe a amplitude da especialidade, visando
o interêsse e a seleção de élites médicas para a mesma; 3) trabalho junto as
organizações hospitalares, no sentido de obter condições de trabalho seguras
e enfermagem treinada nos problemas ligados a anestesia; 4) trabalho de
esclarecimento junto aos cirurgioes, clínicos e especialistas em geral, no
sentido de proporcionar-lhes conhecimento de problemas básicos de
anestesia; 5) formação de anestesistas através da residencia no pós-grado,
e de pessoal auxiliar de enfermagem.

No que diz respeito a uma definição e padronização de títulos e conceitos,
tais como professor, departamento, serviço, cátedra, parece-nos que a situação é confusa em todo o território nacional, não sómente em relação á
anestesia, mas práticamente em todas as Faculdades de Medicina e no
currículo médico. A Lei de Diretrizes e Bases que regulamentou o ensino
em todo o país em 1962, bàsicamente deu autonomia as congregações das
Facultades de Medicina no que diz respeito a sua vida interna. Existe ainda
entretanto controvérsia entre as leis federais, os regulamentos da Universi-
dades, os regimentos das Faculdades, no que diz respeito ao enquadramento
de cargos, funções, hierarquia, direitos e deveres, estando nesta época em
estudo, em todo o território nacional, o Estatuto do Professor Universitário, pretendendo ter jurisdição de ambito nacional.

Em nosso Estado, como resultante de nosso trabalho na Faculdade de
Medicina de Porto Alegre, no presente ano, a anestesiologia passou a ser
oficialmente uma disciplina do currículo médico. Deverá, como disciplina,
integrar um departamento de ensino, o Departamento de Cirurgia, junta-
mente e em igualdade de condicoes com outras disciplinas. No que diz
respeito ao atendimento clínico-hospitalar, constituir-se em departamento
hospitalar, autonomo em seu funcionamento, mantendo vínculos médicos
e administrativos respectivamente com as direções clínica e administrativa
do hospital, e trabalhando em coordinação com as demais clínicas, serviços
e departamentos. Nosso trabalho, em escala reduzida, tem procurado seguir
o que tem sido preconizado pelos centros convencionais do ensino da anestesia, adaptando-se as possibilidades e realidades locais, e estruturado como
segue: 1) organização no presente momento com seis anos de atividade, de
um núcleo pilôto, procurando estruturar em pequenha escala um Departamento de Anestesia Universitário, com seus diferentes setores e funções, nos
seus múltiplos aspectos humanos e técnicos; 2) complementação das ativi-
dades desse núcleo através de locais e serviços qualificados não universitários;
3) participação e colaboração com cátedras e departamentos de ensino;
estágios em anestesia para alunos do curso médico das últimas séries;
4) cursos de divulgação e orientação básica para alunos, através de Centros
Acadêmicos; 5) divulgação, orientação e aulas para enfermeiras nas escolas
de enfermagem; 6) finalmente, formação de especialistas através da residencia ãn pós-graduação.

Nesi: Muchas gracias. Dr. POULSEN, por favor.

Poulsen: I have no intention to give a repetition of my paper from yesterday, in which I tried to explain the present status of anaesthesiology in Denmark. So, I should like to restrict myself and give some comments on some problems we have all over the Scandinavian countries, when we are talking about our specialty. I should like to point out to you that the Scandinavian countries are quite different. That means that my own country, Denmark, is a small country with quite a lot of population per square mile. This is not the same condition we have in Sweden, Norway or Finland. And the problems are, consequently, different in these countries, when we are talking about hospital service. But one thing is to be said to be common in our countries, and that is that, owing to the rapid growth of the population and the nation as a whole, we are always short of manpower. We have a full occupation for everyone, and that means that we await always, and that goes for the hospitals too, have a permanent shortage of personnel, doctors, nurses and so on, mainly due to the fact that our public health system gives free treatment for every person in the nation, on an insurance bases, free treatment in hospitals, free treatment in general practice and so on. This shortage of physicians is important when we are considering the development of a new speciality in a country. Because, if you want to attract the qualified doctors, in a new specialty, you must be able to offer them conditions which are at least not worse than the conditions they can be offered in other specialties. And this made it important that we, in our countries, got an independent status compared with the other specialties. Every other colleague, from other specialties, understood that, and that is the reason why we so quickly gained complete independence and equality regarding economy and so on, with for instance surgery and intern medicine.

The shortage of physicians is going to stay for some years and that is mainly due to the fact that we do not want to lessen the claims for the training. We want still to see that all anaesthetists have a considerable amount of knowledge; besides the direct knowledge of anaesthesiology, they must have a considerable amount of knowledge outside the specialty, that means for intern medicine, surgery and so on. Because the idea has been, during the last ten years, to widen the scope of anaesthesiology in our countries, to take up other tasks than those who are presented to us in the operating room. I am now talking about the nonsurgical field of our daily work, that field which covers all patients with respiratory insufficiencies, coming from various services of the Hospital, and so on.

One problem I should like to mention to you and I think it is found out over the world, is the problem with the small, non-specialised hospital services. And that goes specially for those countries where you have a scattered population over a large area; in such places you will have to have

– and you won't always have – small hospitals with far distances from the nearest larger hospital where specialty services can be found. And I guess the same applies to all the world, that it is extremely difficult to persuade a smaller city, a smaller town, to give up their own hospital and instead of that move their patients to the larger city, which is maybe 1500 miles away. The same problem we have as a matter of fact. And this is one of the problems which will face new specialties like anaesthesiology, radiology and so on. You will always in those smaller services find surgeons – and in some of them may be a single internist – who is able to take care of the patient there, but it is difficult to persuade an anaesthetist to go to such smaller services, mainly due to the fact that the facilities offered to them, regarding to the patient they are going to treat, are not as interesting as they will be in the teaching centers. And that is the reason why we, even in our countries, will find that the physicians have a tendency to accumulate around the teaching centers, universities and so on, and not want to go out. As to the economy, I think that there is nothing to add to what I said yesterday. The only thing to be said in that respect is that the amount of private income in our countries is going down; that goes for surgeons, internists and anaesthetists too. But anyway, we are going in the same bad direction, downwards in that way. Thank you.

Nesi: Muchas gracias, Dr. POULSEN. Es bueno que él nos haya hablado tan claramente de los problemas menos fáciles de la organización hospitalaria. Desde el martes pasado estamos oyendo descripciones de Departamentos de Anestesia ideales; algunos se me figuran casi como organizaciones utópicas. Los que conocemos la realidad de muchos países que se encuentran en distintos grados de evolución y de desarrollo social y económico, sabemos que esos modelos no son fácilmente realizables.

Puesto que todo lo que se ha dicho hasta ahora podría servir más bien para señalar objetivos a ser alcanzados, y como no es necesario insistir sobre las ventajas y sobre todo lo bueno que puede dar un buen Departamento de Anestesia a la ciencia, al hospital y a la comunidad, veamos más bien la situación real de muchos países y las soluciones que se pueden intentar mientras tanto. Felizmente algo nos dijo ya el Dr. LÓPES SOARES, el martes, respecto a soluciones no alcanzadas en Portugal; también el Dr. DE FREITAS BRANDAO explicó con toda franqueza algunas dificultades afrontadas en un país grande y adelantado, y ahora el Dr. POULSEN nos refiere ciertos problemas que existen en hospitales que no son los universitarios o los grandes centros de enseñanza e investigación.

Como bien decía uno de los autores de trabajos presentados en las sesiones previas, las posibilidades de organización dependen fundamentalmente de las estructuras y sistemas asistenciales de cada país. En Anestesiología no es posible crear por iniciativa individual un centro aislado, sin relación con el grado de desarrollo alcanzado por las otras especialidades médicas y sin tomar en cuenta las condiciones físicas y funcionales del ambiente asistencial.

Veamos entonces qué pasos se deben dar y qué caminos se pueden seguir para lograr una situación satisfactoria. Como están en la sala varios de los que han presentado contribuciones al tema, yo quisiera invitarlos a intervenir en la discusión. Empezaré invitando a un representante de la Argentina, país en el cual la Anestesiología comenzó a desarrollarse algunos años antes que en otros que hoy cuentan con organizaciones modelos, como Austria y Dinamarca. Se diría que, en cierto modo, los países que empezaron a organizar sus cuadros de anestesiólogos antes de la segunda guerra, han sido menos afortunados que los que comenzaron después. Tal vez el secreto del éxito de éstos sea precisamente el haber organizado la Anestesiología dentro de sistemas asistenciales más modernos y eficientes. Si el Dr. González Varela nos hace el favor, me gustaría que, muy brevemente, nos explicase cuáles son las dificultades actuales en la República Argentina.

Gonzáles Varela: No desconocemos los graves problemas asistenciales de la Anestesiología en muchos lugares alejados de las grandes ciudades y donde la extensión y la diseminación de la población son muy grandes. Esto es una preocupación constante de la Asociación Argentina de Anestesiología, compartida por las autoridades sanitarias del país. Sabemos que allí los resultados quirúrgicos son muchas veces malos, y que podrían ser mejorados con la preparación adecuada del personal a cargo de la asistencia médica. En muchas ocasiones hemos intervenido en el análisis de estos problemas, tratando de influir sobre las autoridades competentes, a través de entidades médicas y colegios médicos, para que se busquen los medios más elementales que puedan mejorar ese aspecto de la asistencia médica.

Pensamos que se podría contribuir a reducir grandemente la morbilidad y la mortalidad en esos lugares apartados, si los médicos, técnicos y el personal idóneo en algunos casos, fuera adiestrado en los métodos elementales de reanimación, incluso la de recién-nacidos y la de los casos con insuficiencia respiratoria; y si les enseñaran los conocimientos más elementales de la anestesia y los factores de seguridad en el manejo de esos aparatos antiguos, como el de Ombrédanne, que aún se usan en los pequeños hospitales de la campaña.

Como recurso transitorio, hasta que se disponga de especialistas en tales lugares, las entidades médicas de nuestra especialidad debieran buscar el auspicio de las autoridades sanitarias locales para organizar pequeños cursos de perfeccionamiento en esos medios, destinados principalmente a difundir los métodos elementales que hemos mencionado.

Nesi: Muchas gracias. Veo en el Dr. Gonzáles Varela una inclinación muy noble a extender la enseñanza de la Anestesiología a los medios necesitados de la campaña. Este criterio ha sido discutido muchas veces, sobre todo en países latino-americanos, donde se han señalado algunos riesgos de ese tipo de enseñanza elemental y de esa política educacional no selectiva. Los riesgos, en realidad, se podrían reducir a uno sólo: el de mantener detenida la evolución profesional de la especialidad o la formación de médicos anestesiólogos calificados. De todas maneras, considero que esa proyección de la enseñanza, contemplando los intereses de la comunidad y de la especialidad, es una parte de la función que deben cumplir los Departamentos de Anestesiología de los grandes centros. Si tenemos tiempo, vamos a volver sobre este punto, porque merece ser discutido más detenidamente.

Cuando el Dr. POULSEN comentaba la organización en Dinamarca, habló de hospitales medianos y pequeños, en los que, aparentemente, no hay grandes Departamentos de Anestesia como los que tienen los hospitales universitarios. Yo quisiera pedir al Dr. POULSEN que nos explique un poco más detalladamente cómo se trabaja en esos hospitales.

Poulsen: Oh, yes, indeed! As mentioned yesterday, we have at the moment 75 specialists of anaesthesiology in our country. And about a similar number under training. These anaesthetists are able to cover the most immediate needs all over the country, even in the smaller hospitals. But this means that we, in many places, will have to have an anaesthetist working at the same time in two or three hospitals with, say, 20 miles distance from each other, or something like that. This can work, and it works everyday. But I don't think it is a satisfactory working condition to put the anaesthetist to. At least not for a longer period of time. Because this makes him – outside that hospital where he is staying, which is his center – that makes him the assistant of the surgeon in the other hospitals. And he will be unable, in the planetary smaller hospital which he is covering, to carry out his tasks outside the operating room in the same way as he will be able to do it in the hospital which is really his standing place. And this, I think, is extremely unsatisfactory. And we will have to find a way out of this, and the only way to do that will be to force the smaller hospitals to resign in our countries and to concentrate them in some way so that we at least can have a department working with, say, three specialist anaesthetists working together. They will be able to cover up the service twenty-four hours a day and to have a satisfactory working condition.

Nesi: Muchas gracias, Dr. POULSEN. ¿Algún otro Miembro del Panel desea hacer comentarios sobre este punto? Bueno, si nadie lo hace, iremos ubicando dentro del plan de discusión que hemos trazado, algunas preguntas que nos están llegando. Nos habíamos propuesto tratar las normas generales de organización, y aunque considero imposible dar un modelo o un esquema que pueda ser copiado por todos los países, me parece que se pueden discutir los principios básicos de organización. Con ésto se relaciona una de las preguntas. Como lo primordial para la organización es disponer de personal especializado, el Dr. VENKATA RAO, de India, pregunta: ¿Cómo se atraen a los jóvenes médicos hacia la especialidad? Según su experiencia, las dificultades son de orden económico, de orden social y de orden profesional, en cuanto se relaciona con la dependencia del médico especializado al cirujano. Es decir, parecería, que estas tres condiciones hacen menos aceptable, o menos atractiva la especialidad en comparación con algunas otras dentro de la profesión médica. En Dinamarca, según tengo entendido, una manera de conseguir médicos fué la de organizar el Curso Internacional de Anestesiología. Yo quisiera preguntarle al Dr. POULSEN si se observó alguna diferencia en la disponibilidad de médicos inclinados a seguir la especialidad desde que se inauguraron los cursos internacionales, con respecto a la situación que prevalecía antes de comenzar estos cursos.

Poulsen: It is quite clear that as soon as you increase the quality of the training in a certain specialty, this will attract the qualified people. And there is no doubt that the W.H.O. course in Denmark, together with the later started short post-graduate courses given by the Danish Society and by the Scandinavian Society of Anaesthesiologists, that they have meant quite a lot in attracting people, giving them the better possibility of inside the country to get sufficient training, to be, I should say, in a fair competition to the surgeons. Even an old specialty in our countries like intern medicine – we anaesthetists often call them a bit dull in that respect because they thought that everyone could read about intern medicine – and even those have now started post-graduate courses following the lines laid out by the anaesthetists. Because they are afraid not to be able to attract the people they want in the future.

Nesi: Dr. BIANCHETTI, ¿Cómo hacen en Torino para conseguir suficiente número de médicos para constituir un Departamento de Anestesia?

Bianchetti: A Turin nous avons cherché de résoudre le problème invitant les étudiants de médecine pendant le cours normal de médecine et de chirurgie à fréquenter notre clinique. Nous faisons des expérimentations, nous faisons des démonstrations, et nous tenons des leçons aux étudiants, cherchant de leur expliquer les méthodes que nous employons, et les invitant a fréquenter même les salles opératoires de façon qu'ils peuvent se rendre compte de l'importance de l'anesthésie, et qu'ils peuvent se rendre compte du gran besoin que nous avons de jeunes qui se dédient à l'anaesthésie, même si cette discipline est, éventuellement, très fatigante.

Nesi: Muchas gracias. En todo Departamento de Anestesia, casi sin excepción, trabajan enfermeras auxiliares, las cuales – creo que en ésto todos estamos de acuerdo – desarrollan una función importante. Sin embargo, no hemos visto una delimitación definida en las responsabilidades de estas enfermeras, según los relatos que hemos escuchado antes de esta reunión. Sería interesante saber, por lo menos, las funciones y las limitaciones que tienen las enfermeras auxiliares de anestesia en los países que están representados en esta Mesa. El Dr. DE FREITAS BRANDAO, por ejemplo, podría explicarnos las normas que rigen en su propio hospital o en su propio Departamento de Anestesia. ¿Qué se espera de las enfermeras y qué es lo que se les permite hacer?

de Freitas Brandao: Básicamentes lhes está proibida, em todo o território nacional, a realização de anestesias. Quer dizer, o que lhes é permitido fazer, e o trabalho ao qual nós nos referimos aqui, consiste num trabalho de divulgação, de situação e de orientação a essas funções que o Dr. NESI pergunta, e que, a meu entender, são as seguintes: inicialmente, um conhecimento de todos os problemas do anestesista em uma sala de cirugia; que dizer, qual o papel que devem representar no sentido de auxílio na indução de uma anestesia, na recuperação imediata de uma anestesia, quais os problemas em que vão também axuliá-lo na recuperação pós-anestésica imediata, eu disse, tarefas inerentes a sua função de enfermagem e, básicamente, funções todas elas auxiliares, caracterizadas por uma proibição de execução de anestesias.

Nesi: Muchas gracias. Dr. IWATSUKI, ¿Qué hacen las enfermeras de anestesia en Sendai?

Iwatsuki: We have now 3 anaesthesia nurses. They may help a doctor for giving anaesthesia in the operating room, but mostly they work in the recovery room. And we don't allow nurses to give any anaesthesia.

Bianchetti: Il faut dire avant tout qu'en Italie, jusqu'à présent nous n'avons pas d'infirmières anesthésistes. La question donc n' apas été discutée, mais nous croyons que seulement les anesthésistes qualifiés peuvent donner des anesthésies.

Poulsen: Well, it seems that I am quite alone on one side of the field of the battle. At least when we are talking about nurses. An maybe it is a kind of an unpopular point-of-view I am bringing forward. But let me put it in this way: I hate the word "nurse-anaesthetist" or "anaesthesia-nurse". What we have in our countries, is nurses in the department of anaesthesiology; this means that there are no prohibitions for them to do anything *except* what is prohibited by their chief. As their chief will always be the Head of the Department, which means, and anaesthetist. Never a surgeon or anyone else. We do not have any State Laws telling that nurses are not allowed to give anaesthesia, or something like that. Because if a nurse is acting, and that is independant of if, it is an action inside the recovery room, where a patient suddenly gets a cardiac stand-still – and as we went – *she* has to carry on artificial ventilation and extern cardiac massage until the physician arrives; whatever she does; that goes for small anaesthetics too, if you may permit me the phrase "small anaesthetic" here just for one second. She is acting completely under the responsibility of the physician who has put her into charge. The general trend in our countries is of course to let the nurses help the physicians in performing their work. To make it easier for us to work, and to widen our field of work, which means to give us the possibility to treat more patients better than we would do if we would have to do these things alone – or my be let the junior surgeons perform the job, as it was done twenty years ago in our countries. Being a young medical student, I acted as an assistant in surgery. I didn't know anything about anaesthesia. The first day I entered an operating room, I was put in charge of the anaesthetic. It is peculiar, I am still an anaesthetist . . . But I guess the surgeons had the responsibility for what happened in that particular case. As a matter of fact, I think it is better to have well-trained nurses working under the responsibility of the physician-anaesthetist, than it is to have young unexperienced surgeons doing a job they don't like to do and which they are not at all qualified to do.

Nesi: Muchas gracias, Dr. POULSEN. ¿Hay alguien de la Mesa que quiera discutir las observaciones del Dr. POULSEN? No. Yo quisiera plantearle un caso particular al Dr. BIANCHETTI. En un buen hospital de Torino, con un buen Departamento de Anestesia y con excelente personal de médicos anestesiólogos, el Dr. BIANCHETTI hace una anestesia raquídea para una operación prolongada de abdomen. La operación dura tres horas. ¿Quién permanece en la cabecera del enfermo vigilándolo durante esas tres horas?

Bianchetti: Chez nous, sera toujours l'anesthésiste qui a pratiqué la rachidienne qui restera à la tête d'un malade. Nous cherchons de ne laisser presque jamais du personnel non qualifié près du malade.

Nesi: Muchas gracias. Antes de seguir adelante, si alguien del público quiere hacer algún comentario o crítica sobre este punto en particular, yo lo invito cordialmente a que haga uso del podio. Si no es así, pasaremos a otro punto.

En estos días se ha hablado mucho de Departamentos Autónomos, pero creo que para muchos no está muy claro el concepto de autonomía en este terreno. Me parece que vale la pena discutir un poco este concepto, para evitar cualquier error de interpretación en el público y en los que lean las Actas de esta Mesa Redonda. ¿Dr. DE FREITAS BRANDAO, no querría usted hacer un comentario sobre Autonomía?

de Freitas Brandao: Me parece que nunca deverá ser esquecida a natureza da especialidade, e que na maior parte das veses, o trabalho do anestesista representa um meio para ser atingido um fim. Eu penso, no que diz respeito a situação hospitalar, e na qualidade de departamento, os de anestesia deverão ter uma situação identica aos demais departamentos e serviços hospitalares, ou seja, subordinação direta a direção clínica do hospital, subordinação indireta as administraçoes hospitalares, e trabalho em coordenação con tôdas as demais clínicas e servicos.

Nesi: Muchas gracias, Dr. de Freitas. ¿ Hay alguien más en el Panel que quiera comentar sobre autonomía ? No. Yo creo que, a veces, se incurre en un error de concepto cuando se habla de las funciones y responsabilidades del Departamento. Para muchos parecería que el Departamento de Anestesia es una sección privilegiada, y entienden por autonomía, una especie de independencia absoluta en el manejo y atención de los pacientes. Uno de los puntos en discusión, el que se refiere a las funciones, obligaciones y responsabilidades del Departamento de Anestesia, se relaciona estrechamente con la interpretación de la autonomía del Departamento. Hoy mismo se presentaba la descripción de uno de esos departamentos que me parecen demasiado idealizados, y se hablaba de la consulta pre-anestésica en forma tal, que parecería que el enfermo ingresa en el Departamento de Anestesia para ser estudiado y diagnosticado, para indicar su tratamiento y su operación. No quedaría más que llamar al cirujano para operarlo.

Esta mañana, el Dr. Callegari, ha descripto un sistema de consulta pre-anestésica, según es cual parecería que hasta los exámenes de laboratorio son ordenados por el Departamento de Anestesia. Está muy bien que el anestesiólogo intervenga en el estudio pre-operatorio del paciente, pero no creo que deba hacerlo independientemente de los servicios médicos de un hospital bien organizado. El hospital debe tener un sistema perfectamente coordinado para el estudio médico del enfermo y éste debe ir a la operación con una historia clínica bien hecha, en cuya elaboración podría participar el anestesiólogo. Pero me parece exagerado que el anestesiólogo deba rehacer la historia, bajo el pretexto de cumplir esa función tan importante, que es el estudio pre-anestésico del paciente. Como he nombrado al Dr. Callegari, yo le voy a pedir que aclare un poco su criterio personal, después de los comentarios de algunos de los Miembros del Panel.

Poulsen: I should very much like to comment upon this. My very poor understanding of Spanish, made it impossible for me to distinguish between the words "should be" or "should have", and the word "had", this morning when Dr. Callegari spoke. He talked about the Department, and I got the impression that he meant that this was the ideal department which he wanted to build, and so on and so forth. But I did not really get it, because, afterwards, our very honoured Chairman said that he congratulated him because he has such and such a department. You see, it is just language difficulties ... Maybe I should like to bring forward one point. I think it is important here. And that is: we must never forget that the patients, they come to the hospital because they have an illness, and they want to be cured of that illness. I am not quite sure that many patients come to the hospital to please us, just because they like to be sleeping sometime and have an anaesthetic. And as a matter of fact, this is really a thing which makes it quite clear where our position will be, in the total structure of the hospital. It will always be in the middle, as a department of service to the other departments. So, speaking about autonomy and independence and all that, I think we are getting on a dangerous road, where we might easily get off the road and fall into the side of the road. Let us try to get back again and just say: we have, in our specialty, a service to offer to the patient. We can make the surgery possible, we can help our colleagues in the non-surgical services, in the treatment of their patients. And in some few cases, the patients, in the true sense of the word, belong to us. I am now talking about poisoning cases, cases, say, with drowning, other cases, primarily needing resuscitation. Because everyone of you will agree that we are anaesthetists and "emergensiologists" at the same time. But in most cases, we are a man between the surgeons on one side, and the internist on the other side. Let us keep to that road. Let us be the heads of the Intensive Care Units, because this is a meeting for the different specialties. And let us stay there in collaboration and very good common work with the other colleagues, and never try to get complete independence. Let me put it quite bluntly: *No* specialist, in any specialty, is independent today. Because specialization means absolute necessity for cooperation if the right and the best results are to be achieved.

Nesi: Muchas gracias, Dr. POULSEN. Lo felicito por la claridad con que ha expresado la idea que, seguramente, compartimos la mayor parte de nosotros. ¿Hay alguien de la Mesa que quiera discutir el mismo punto? No. ¿El Dr. CALLEGARI sería tan amable en comentar este punto?

Callegari: Primeramente tendría que referirme al sentido de la autonomía del Departamento de Anestesiología. Entendemos por autonomía, el hecho de no estar debajo de otro departamento, sino a la misma altura que el resto de los departamentos en la organización hospitalaria. Si es una organización vertical la que existe en el hospital, estaremos debajo de la Dirección o del Comité Directivo, y dependiendo solamente de ellos. Esto, en cuanto concierne a la organización hospitalaria. Pero si nos referimos ahora a la atención del paciente, en ningún momento, al menos así lo entiendo, podemos estar disgregados o separados de los otros departamentos o servicios del hospital. Tenemos que colaborar con ellos, porque solamente dependemos del paciente. Entonces hay dos aspectos: el aspecto de organización hospitalaria, y el aspecto de departamento al servicio del paciente.

En realidad, esta mañana me refería a la organización ideal del Departamento de Anestesiología, no como un sueño, sino en cuanto concierne al entrenamiento y a las enseñanzas que nosotros, los jefes de Departamentos de Anestesiología, debemos inculcar en los residentes y en el personal que está haciendo su entrenamiento técnico. No es que deseamos hacer el preanestésico sin valorar el diagnóstico con que el paciente va a la operación. No. Nuestro estudio pre-anestésico tampoco se hace con igual intensidad en todos los pacientes. Si me he referido en forma amplia al estudio preanestésico que debe llevar a cabo el Departamento de Anestesiología, no quise significar que debe comprender a todos los pacientes o desconocer el diagnóstico clínico y operatorio. Simplemente quiero decir que en el aspecto de investigación y el aspecto de enseñanza debemos estar preparados para realizar este estudio en tal o cual paciente que llega a la sala de operaciones, y que ese estudio debe estar dirigido especialmente a los residentes en entrenamiento. Nosotros compartimos la idea de que no solamente en aspecto anestesiológico debemos atender a los pacientes, sino en todos los aspectos que conciernen al paciente dentro de la unidad operatoria.

Nesi: Muchas gracias. Bueno, con estas palabras del Dr. CALLEGARI vemos un poco más claramente su concepto, el que tal vez yo no comprendí muy bien esta mañana. Parece que es principalmente la función docente del Departamento, la que obliga a intensificar, y tal vez a exagerar un poco, la intervención del Departamento en el estudio pre-operatorio del paciente. Me gustaría escuchar ahora al Dr. VÁZQUEZ, de Argentina.

Vázquez: Si me permiten, quisiera hacer unas muy breves consideraciones a propósito de un punto que ya ha sido tocado: la manera más efectiva de atraer a nuestra especialidad al joven recién-graduado, al que tiene sanas aspiraciones, es decir el material más propicio para desarrollar. No al médico que ha andado de un lado a otro, que ha fracasado o que no ha conseguido hacer un patrimonio y que piensa en la anestesia como un medio de ganar dinero de una manera más fácil y más rápida. Quiero explicar entonces, el punto de vista argentino que, hasta cierto punto, es bastante uniforme.

Nosotros creemos que el gran factor de atracción, el más firme y el más difícil de conseguir, es el jerarquizar nuestra especialidad. Para que sea una especialidad realmente médica, es necesario que el anestesiólogo del hospital esté realmente integrado al hospital, que esté permanente, realmente conectado con el resto de los médicos. No que sea un hombre que viene cinco minutos antes para dormir a un enfermo que no ha examinado el día anterior. Que no concurre a los ateneos ni a las conferencias, que no va a los comités, que no puede evacuar ninguna consulta porque no tiene conocimientos básicos, y que solamente conoce una técnica: protóxido, un relajante, un barbiturato, y no hay quién lo saque de eso. Al que alguna vez ha tenido la idea de ir a la Anestesiología, debemos demostrarle, por el contrario, que va a seguir siendo médico. Porque lo que aleja a mucha gente, es pensar que por ser anestesista dejará de ser médico, y porque muchos profanos creen todavía que el anestesista puede o no ser médico. No. Nosotros creemos que el que se inicia en anestesia debe tener la firme convicción de que, por el resto de su vida, va a ser un buen médico, perfectamente integrado al resto de la medicina. Y ahí está la igualdad jerárquica. Esa es nuestra fuerza. Ese es el fundamento de la autonomía y ese es el punto de vista argentino.

Ahora bien, ¿cuál es el modo de alcanzar esa meta? Lenta, pero de manera firme, ir calificando gente, con buenos y verdaderos cursos de enseñanza. Reales cursos de enseñanza, en los que se tengan no solamente planes, o proyectos muy plausibles, pero teóricos o para el futuro, sino *Resultados*. Por eso yo me permito solicitar al coordinador del Panel que pida a aquéllos que me han precedido en el uso de la palabra, que en lo posible, hablen de sus resultados concretos en lo que se refiere a la enseñanza. Muchas gracias.

Nesi: Muchas gracias, Dr. VÁZQUEZ. Voy a seguir su consejo, pero antes me gustaría oir al Dr. POULSEN. ¿Algún comentario sobre lo que dijo el Dr. VÁZQUEZ?

Poulsen: This brings me to another question which has been brought up here by Dr. STEINHAUS, from the U.S.A., who asked what aspects of anaesthesiology really attracts the medical students who select anaesthesiology as their specialty in our country. And I really feel that Dr. VÁZQUEZ has touched upon an *extremely* important matter. The question is: how do we get the best of the medical students? And what is it really what can make this specialty more attractive than other ones? I should make it quire clear and say that, in our country, there is no doubt that the participation in the resuscitative field of the anaesthetist is being the most important point in that respect. In our countries the medical students have to pass two terms of lectures and courses in anaesthesiology, before their final examination and graduation as medical doctors. And it is my feeling that the general items about giving anaesthesia, and all that, cannot compete in our country with the privilege of being allowed to use a knife on a patient. But there is no doubt that they are very interested as soon as we get into talking about the insufficient respiration, circulation, the resuscitation, and so on and so forth. This has even made it possible for us to make it necessary, for every specialist in surgery, that he, at this moments, shall serve at least one year in a Department of Anaesthesiology as a resident, before he is recognized a specialist in surgery. And thus, those who primarily were attracted by surgery, they switched over and went on in anaesthesiology, because they found this was more interesting.

Nesi: Muchas gracias, Dr. Poulsen. ¿Alguien quiere discutir ese punto? Se ha hablado muchas veces de tratamiento de insuficiencia respiratoria, reanimación respiratoria, y todas esas funciones que actualmente, en buenos Departamentos, se llevan a cabo en Unidades de Terapia Intensiva, o en Salas de Recuperación. Este parece ser un ideal que en muchos sitios, todavía no se ha podido llevar a efecto. Yo creo que la dificultad más grande para conseguirlo es el sistema de trabajo. Creo que debiéramos aclarar, para comprendernos mejor entre nosotros, que no es en todas partes que el médico anestesiólogo concurre diariamente a un hospital determinado y permanece en ese hospital desde la mañana hasta las horas de la tarde. Y creo que es necesario aclarar ésto para que se comprenda por qué no siempre es posible organizar una Sala de Recuperación que sea a la vez un centro de tratamiento de enfermos graves, por condiciones respiratorias o circulatorias. Por experiencia propia, puedo afimar que es imposible pensar en la organización de estos servicios auxiliares de la Anestesiología, mientras no haya una estructura básica adecuada y mientras el personal, no sólo el personal médico sino también el auxiliar, no esté organizado en forma tal, que pueda cumplir a cabalidad esta función, para mostrar resultados que puedan inducir a nuestros colegas médicos y cirujanos a enviar enfermos a esas unidades.

No son sólo las facilidades físicas, arquitectónicas o estructurales, las que más importan. Lo esencial, a mi modo de ver, es el sistema de trabajo del personal. Casi todos los que estamos hablando en este Panel tenemos la suerte de trabajar en hospitales universitarios, donde se cuentan con facilidades de personal y con facilidades de equipos que nos han permitido organizar, en distintas formas, servicios auxiliares de este tipo. Pero en otros hospitales de otras ciudades, aún de nuestros propios países o en otros países del mundo, ésto no ha podido ser realizado todavía.

A los que esperan organizar servicios de este tipo, quisiera aclararles que nosotros, en nuestro hospital, no pretendemos que el anestesiólogo sea el único que entiende de estos problemas. El no reemplaza al neumonólogo o al cardiólogo, por ejemplo, sino que colabora con ellos aplicando procedimientos que emplea habitualmente en Cirugía. Creo que es importante dejar este punto aclarado para que sea más fácil introducir la idea en hospitales donde no existe todavía este sistema de trabajo, para convencer a los otros colegas, especialistas en otras ramas de la Medicina, qué es lo que nosotros podemos darles, qué es lo que ellos pueden esperar de nosotros, y en qué forma deseamos cooperar con ellos en el tratamiento de estos enfermos.

Las necesidades y las funciones del Departamento en hospitales universitarios son un tanto distintas de las de otros hospitales donde la enseñanza no es la función esencial. Se explica así, que en los hospitales universitarios hayan dependencias, hayan funciones y responsabilidades que no son esenciales en otros hospitales. Incluyo en estas consideraciones un aspecto de que se habla con cierta frecuencia: la organización de un laboratorio anexo al Departamento de Anestesia. En nuestro hospital, en nuestro Departamento de Anestesia, tenemos un laboratorio, pero no creo que sea necesario en todo hospital y bajo todas las condiciones. En un hospital bien organizado debe haber un laboratorio para análisis de emergencia post-y pre-operatoria, y para los que se necesiten durante la operación, el cual no necesariamente tiene que estar bajo la dependencia del Departamento de Anestesia o de los anestesiólogos. No se puede pretender que todo anestesiólogo, por ser tal, esté obligado a dominar técnicas de laboratorio. Lo que sí debemos esperar de ellos, es que sepan interpretar resultados de laboratorio. El laboratorio es útil en la enseñanza, no sólo como recurso didáctico para ampliar el campo de la enseñanza, incluso para enseñar los detalles de ciertas técnicas que luego puedan ser empleadas en investigación por los que asisten a esos departamentos con fines de entrenamiento.

Si alguno de los Miembros de la Mesa está en desacuerdo con mi opinión, yo le ruego que me lo haga saber; lo mismo, si alguien quiere agregar algún comentario a lo que estoy diciendo. Como nadie dice nada, yo voy a pedirle al Dr. Iwatsuki, que nos explique cuál es la función del Departamento de Anestesia en Sendai, en reanimación y en tratamiento de insuficiencias respiratorias. Desearía saber también si ustedes disponen de laboratorio propio.

Iwatsuki: In regard to the laboratory, we have two: one is attached to the hospital, and the other one is attached to our own department. So, if we want to know something about the conditions of the patient, for example, serum electrolytes, liver functions or something like that, we can obtain the data from the central laboratory of the hospital. And if we want to know some special data, particularly for the purpose of research, we can do it in our own laboratory. We have not yet a so-called well equipped intensive care unit. Therefore, if we have such a case, then we treat the patient in the recovery room, or in the ward under collaboration of the doctors in charge. An intensive care unit seems very important not only for the treatment of patients, but also for the activity of anaesthesiologists.

Nesi: Este último punto que toca el Dr. Iwatsuki, me parece que es importante para los que esperan tener algún día una Unidad de Terapia Intensiva. Yo creo que el mejor camino para demostrar a las autoridades administrativas del hospital y a los otros servicios del hospital, la utilidad de una unidad de terapia intentensiva, es comenzar a prestar ese servicio en la propia sala de recuperación. La Sala de Recuperación casi no necesita ser modificada para prestar servicios como Unidad de Terapia Intensiva.

Como el Dr. Iwatsuki mencionó también el laboratorio como centro de investigación, yo creo que también hay algunos errores de concepto cuando se dice que todo Departamento de Anestesia tiene tres funciones que cumplir: una asistencial, otra de enseñanza y otra de investigación. Creo que se sobreestima un poco el concepto de la tercera función, la de investigación. En mi propio Departamento – que es el de un hospital universitario – me gusta hablar más bien de *estudio*, que de investigación. Yo preparo a mis colaboradores para el estudio, como un camino para llegar a la investigación. Los trabajos serios de investigación probablemente irán surgiendo a medida que se van desarrollando estos estudios, pero nuestra finalidad inmediata no es inventar nada nuevo. Se repite, incluso lo que se ha hecho en otros centros, nada más que como una disciplina de estudio, como un entrenamiento y como un medio de ir seleccionando a los más aptos, a los más capaces, a los que probablemente serán después auténticos investigadores científicos.

Muchos Departamentos tienen la suerte de contar con laboratorios propios para la investigación. Algunos de estos Departamentos han llegado a convertirse en verdaderos Institutos de Anestesiología. Yo pienso que, si bien ésto es ideal y mejor así si uno lo consigue, no puede considerárselo como indispensable para realizar trabajos de investigación. Cuando se tiene la suerte de trabajar cerca de Institutos de Fisiología, de Farmacología y de otras ciencias básicas de la Universidad, ¿por qué no recurrir a esos laboratorios, aprovechando sus equipos y personal técnico, en vez de esperar la creación de un nuevo laboratorio para recién empezar a investigar? Para obtener la colaboración de aquellos institutos y departamentos de enseñanza, hay que demostrarles, en primer lugar, los beneficios que puede aportarles el anestesiólogo que es, a la vez, un estudioso.

La investigación más accesible al anestesista, a mi modo de ver, es la investigación clínica. Esto necesita más que una buena disciplina de observación y de interpretación, suficientes conocimientos básicos y tiempo, paciencia y dedicación. Creo que es el camino más fácil, por donde conviene empezar, sin creer que investigación es solamente el estudio que se hace sobre animales en el laboratorio.

Poulsen: Would you mind, please? Our Chairman has an extraordinarily clear and good way of expressing my opinion on this matter; I have no comments.

Nesi: Vamos a pasar a las preguntas. Desgraciadamente, tenemos muchas en la Mesa y ésto nos obligará a cortar un poquito el programa.

El Dr. GHOSE, de Etiopía, pregunta al Dr. BIANCHETTI si no piensa que dos años de entrenamiento en Anestesiología es muy poco. Agrega que, personalmente, él propicia cinco años.

Bianchetti: Oui, j'ai dit que jusqu'à présent le temps de préparation de l'anesthésiste est de deux ans. Pendant ces deux ans, il doit soutenir des examens, des examens très durs. On fait des études d'anatomie, de physiologie, de pharmacologie et une étude des sujets spécialisés: l'anesthésie en O.R.L., en obstétriquegynécologie, etc. Mais j'ai dit, en effet, que nous souhaitons que, dans les prochaines années, la préparation de l'anesthésiste italien soit portée à trois ans. Je pense que, actuellement, presque tous les pays d'Europe sont d'accord sur ce point.

Nesi: ¿Está satisfecho, Dr. GHOSE? El Dr. STEINBERG, de Venezuela, pregunta al Dr. IWATSUKI si considera él una ventaja pertenecer a la Sociedad de Anestesiología sin ser anestesista calificado, y si considera práctico tener un «board», habiendo tantos problemas locales. En fin, si todo ésto no significa una dispersión de esfuerzos.

Iwatsuki: So far, at present, a doctor who is a member of the Society of Anaesthesiology does not have any special privileges. Because the Society of Anaesthesiology embraces all doctors who have interest in the science of anaesthesiology.

Nesi: Un colega de Guanabara pregunta al Dr. DE FREITAS BRANDAO si está prohibido a las enfermeras hacer anestesias en todo el territorio nacional, ¿por qué se les permite hacerlo en ciertos hospitales federales?

de Freitas Brandao: Eu casualmente tenho aqui comigo uma certidão, cuja fotocopia foi feita em 1954. Essa responde especìficamente a esta e outras perguntas semelhantes. A resposta é clara: é flagrantemente ilegal. Por outro lado, em tôda a legislação que regulamentou a execução da profissão de enfermeira, também é especificamente proibido. De modo que me parece que o problema deveria ser encaminhado a Comissão de Etica e Defesa Profissional da nossa Sociedade, a fim de que ela sugerisse as medidas cabíveis e incaminhasse, com a maior fôrça, e com maior possibilidade de solução, o problema específico que me está sendo perguntado.

Nesi: Edison Penna pregunta: En un hospital con funciones de asistencia médica y enseñanza, en que el anestesiólogo es a la vez instructor, qué relación debería haber entre el número de anestesiólogos en funciones y el número de intervenciones quirúrgicas anuales, y qué relación entre anestesiólogos y residentes de Anestesiología?

Es una pregunta un poco difícil, porque todo eso varía mucho de acuerdo a las estructuras y organización en cada país. Paso esta pregunta al Dr. DE FREITAS BRANDAO, porque como el que pregunta es un latino-americano, puede ser que tenga condiciones de trabajo más próximas a las del Brasil.

de Freitas Brandao: Eu não teria elementos para responder ao colega. Talvês a pergunta pudesse ser em relação a êsse tipo de cálculo, feito mais pelos hospitais de São Paulo, especialmente o Hospital de Clínicas, ou talvês pelos hospitais do Rio de Janeiro. Porque, como eu disse aqui inicialmente, todo o nosso trabalho e um trabalho pilóto, em núcleo reduzido, que ainda não teve essa preocupação com êsse tipo de cálculo.

Nesi: Muchas gracias. Hay una pregunta muy interesante del Prof. LARENG, de Toulouse, Francia. Dice que en Francia, de un modo general, el anestesiólogo no puede ser, él solo, responsable de un enfermo, y pregunta si eso está reglamentado en otros sitios. Como no podemos hacer una encuesta universal, nos vamos a tener que conformar con saber cuál es la situación en Italia, en Brasil, en Dinamarca y en Japón. Por eso les preguntaré a los cuatro Miembros del Panel si, en sus respectivos países, se permite al anestesiólogo ser el único reponsable de un enfermo, no solamente durante una operación, sino en una intoxicación barbitúrica, por ejemplo – creo que esa es la idea del Dr. LARENG.

Bianchetti: Ca dépend, si on parle de responsabilité pénale ou bien de responsabilité civile. En Italie, au point de vue de la responsabilité pénale, seulement celui qui pratique une méthode d'anesthésie (et s'il n'entraîne pas l'intervention du chirugien ou d'un autre spécialiste) est le seul responsable. Tandis que du point de vue civil, le responsable dans la plupart des cas, est seulement l'hôpital ou travaille l'anesthésiste.

Nesi: Merci bien. Dr. DE FREITAS BRANDAO?

de Freitas Brandao: Tenho a impressão de que no Brasil, o problema é completamente claro. Quer dizer, o médico anestesista tem assegurados por lei todos os direitos iguais aos outros médicos, é específicamente neste tipo de situação enfocado pelo Prof. NESI, em relação a uma situação de coma, uma situação respiratória, etc., êle tem responsabilidade legal no atendimento que êle fôr prestar sòzinho.

Poulsen: As about the Scandinavia, this is quite clear. Any physician can have the sole responsibility for a given patient. It has been made quite clear by one of our High Court Judges, who has had to pass a sentence about that. He said: "It is without importance to which doctor the patient goes first". So this does mean that no surgeon, or no internist will have a more close connection – legally spoken – to the patient than the anaesthetist.

Iwatsuki: In Japan, anaesthesiologists in the operating room are of course responsible for the patient. And in the post-operative course, the anaesthesiologists are responsible for the time being in regard to the complications which might be due to the anaesthesia itself. And in other cases, for example the barbiturate poisoning, or something like that, when we get the consultation from other doctors, we take care of the patient, in cooperation with the doctors in charge of other departments.

Nesi: Muchas gracias. ¿El Prof. LARENG está satisfecho? ¿Quiere agregar algún comentario? No.

El Dr. OBLADEN pregunta, esta vez al Dr. VÁZQUEZ, si en su país está reglamentada la concesión de título de especialista de Anestesia a extranjeros y cuáles son los requisitos indispensables para obtenerlo.

Vázquez: Como mencioné hace un instante, en nuestro país se viene tomando exámen para extender un Certificado o Diploma de la Asociación Argentina de Anestesiología, hace ya cinco años. Cualquier médico de cualquier país del mundo, que acredite su condición de graduado y que demuestre también de manera fehaciente que ha practicado la especialidad en forma exclusiva, por un período no menor de cinco años, puede dar examen. En diciembre del año 1963, el Presidente de la Sociedad Uruguaya de Anestesiología aprobó ese examen y actualmente ostenta su Diploma. Además estamos ansiosos por contar, por sentirnos honrados con la visita de otros médicos extranjeros que aspiren a nuestro Diploma. Gracias.

Nesi: Muchas gracias, Dr. VÁZQUEZ. El Dr. GONZÁLES TORRES, de Argentina, pregunta si la Federación Mundial de Sociedades de Anestesiología ha tomado contacto con la UNESCO, con la ONU o con la WHO, para conseguir, mediante recomendaciones a los gobiernos, la autonomía de los servicios de Anestesiología. Y si ésto no se ha hecho así, pregunta si los Miembros del Panel no creen que tal cosa sería conveniente. Yo no sé que pensarán los Miembros del Panel, pero como yo también formo parte del mismo, diré que me parece que esto no puede conseguirse mediante reglamentos de orden internacional; que ésto es algo que, dentro de cada país, debe conseguirlo cada Sociedad de Anestesiología. De todas maneras, como hay Miembros en el Panel que tienen más relación con organismos internacionales, voy a pedir a uno de ellos, en particular, el Dr. POULSEN, qué es lo que piensa al respecto.

Poulsen: I do not think as a matter of fact that the World Federation is able to interfere with that proposition that you mentioned, Dr. GONZÁLEZ. But I am quite sure that the World Federation will be able to help the member societies in different ways. One of the ways would be, as it already has

been done, to try to, together with the WHO, to create and support new
and existing teaching centers of anaesthesiology. And secondly, I should
like to mention another matter – which I think is of importance in this
point – and that is that the World Federation has just established now a
Committee. A Committee dealing with an investigation in cardio-pulmo-
nary resuscitation, which is going to be a kind of international questionnaire,
being sent out all over the world, trying to give the anaesthetist in each
country the possibility of being the man ahead dealing with resuscitation.
That might help the policy in each national country. I think these cons-
ultative ways, these ways of impressing upon the single governments, that is
the only we can achieve what we want.

Nesi: Muchas gracias. Hay tres preguntas que, en cierto modo, están
relacionadas, porque se refieren a enseñanza en pre-grado de Medicina – a
estudiantes de Medicina –. Dice el Dr. Alfonso Zuliani, de Río, que en la
Facultad Nacional de Medicina de la Universidad de Brasil, incluyen en el
programa algunas clases de Anestesia, y que procuran enseñar a todos los
estudiantes de los últimos años a intubar y ventilar a los pacientes. Desearía
él saber qué piensan los Miembros del Panel sobre esta orientación.

Al lado de eso, Dr. Barmaimón, de Uruguay, quisiera conocer la opinión
de los Miembros del Panel sobre los estudiantes de Medicina ejerciendo
funciones de anestesista. Y otro dice así: «¿No sería una buena sugerencia
el entrenamiento obligatorio, no ya de los estudiantes, sino de cirujanos y
médicos obstétras, durante algunos pocos meses?». Es decir, los tres se
refieren a entrenamiento, enseñanza y responsabilidades para estudiantes o
médicos que no van a ser necesariamente anestesiólogos.

de Freitas Brandao: Inicialmente, em relação à pergunta relacionada
com o estudante de medicine executando anestesias: Eu tenho a impressão
que não é uma tarefa de estudante. Em relação a pergunta do Dr. Zuliani:
certamente é uma coisa boa e útil e êle, como muitos outros colegas, em uma
série de lugares no Brasil, estão fazendo êsse esfôrço isolado. Me parece que
para expressar un pensamento comum, a responder sumàriamente a tôdas
as perguntas, eu diria que, em relação a ensino, há um acordo mais ou menos
unânime que este ensino deva ser dividido e dirigido nos seguintes pontos:
O ensino curricular, destinado ao estudante de medicina, de formas variadas,
colaborações com departamentos de ensino, com cátedras e ensino informativo; o ensino de pós-graduação, através da residência, um ensino carac-
terìsticamente mais formativo do que informativo, mais de educação do
que de instrução; e finalmente, o ensino e divulgação de conceitos de anestesia em outros servição e departamentos. Responde exatamente àquilo que
foi comentado em relação a cirurgiões, em relação a obstetras, e que acho uma
coisa útil. E, finalmente, o outro setor de ensino a ser trabalhado seria o

setor de enfermagem, com mira específicamente às salas de recuperação, às salas de operação, e a tôdas as técnicas de enfermagem relacionadas com os assuntos de anestesia.

Nesi: Muchas gracias. Temo que sea demasiado tarde, de modo que, desgraciadamente, vamos a tener que dar por terminado este Panel. Yo quiero pedir al público que me disculpe si he tomado la palabra con cierta insistencia y si he hablado más de lo que correspondía a un Presidente de Mesa Redonda. En descargo de mi conciencia, tengo que decirles que lo hice por temor de que, dadas las circunstancias, el tiempo no permitiera discutir puntos importantes de organización. Antes que pasarlos por alto, quise que se conociera, por lo menos, la opinión de una persona que, después de todo, también forma parte del Panel. Más aún, subrayando con cierto énfasis mis puntos de vista personales, traté de incitar al debate, para profundizar el análisis de algunos aspectos controvertibles de nuestro tema.

F. Anaesthesia for cardio-vascular surgery

Chairman: T. Cecil Gray Liverpool
Members: R. V. G. Amaral, Sao Paulo; J. Beard, London; E. Ciocatto,
Turin; M. H. Holmdahl, Uppsala; J. P. Payne, London; G. J. Rees,
Liverpool; B. A. Sellick, London; A. L. Stead, Liverpool; H. Yamamura,
Tokyo; M. Zindler, Düsseldorf.

Zindler reported on changes of cardiac output estimated with the dye dilution (indocyanine green) method in 18 patients undergoing correction of a mitral stenosis in neuroleptanaesthesia using droperidol and phentanyl.

Compared with a control value after premedication with thalamonal the changes of the cardiac index in neuroleptanalgesia were suprisingly small and varied in the average from 96% to 106% until the opening of the thorax.

In contrast to this series in 3 other groups with barbiturate and nitrous oxide, barbiturate, nitrous oxide and ether and barbiturate, nitrous oxide and halothane there was a marked decrease of the cardiac index the lowest values being after opening of the chest between 50% and 58% of the control before induction of anaesthesia.

As to be expected the cardiac index rose markedly in all groups after splitting the mitral stenosis depending on the relief of the stenosis. In the neuroleptanaesthesia group it was considerably higher than in the 3 other groups.

These remarkable differences were no longer seen at the determinations one and three hours postoperatively.

Supportive therapy, ventilation etc. were kept as uniform as possible in all groups. The only difference was a higher dose of curare (24 mg) in the barbiturate – nitrous oxide group as compared to the average of 15,4 mg in the neuroleptanaesthesia group and 14,4 mg in the barbiturate – ether group.

It was concluded that the demonstrated lack of cardiac depression of neuroleptanaesthesia is very valuable in patients with limited cardiac reserve especially in heart operations.

Different methods for determination of cardiac output were discussed by Gray. Not satisfactory for routine use is the method described by Fick, its potential mistakes are considerable. The dye diluting method is more suitable. Determination by transluminating the ear lobe is useful but can only be utilized in patients with vasodilatation and is difficult to evaluate during shock and insufficient blood flow in the carotis externa. In canine experiments HOLMDAHL found that the force of cardiac (atrial) contraction is lessened during halothane anaesthesia. Changes of metabolism (acid-base balance) during extracorporeal circulation were discussed by AMARAL and during hypothermia by YAMAMURA.

Sellick favors the addition of 10% carbon dioxide during hypothermia.

Ciocatto and **Rees** reported about experiences with haemodilution while using the heart-lung machine. Different anesthetic methods for operations with the heart-lung machine were discussed by STEAD, HOLMDAHL and AMARAL.

Sellick recommended leaving the endotracheal tube in place after major operations in patients of poor risk and continuing analgesia with artificial ventilation of 50% nitrous oxide, for some patients up to 24 hours.
1. He had found that considerable advantages could be gained in terms of increased comfort and improved respiratory function if controlled respiration was maintained for 6–18 hours after the completion of major heart surgery. This had been achieved by retaining in situ the oral endotracheal tube and making no attempt to reverse any residual curare.
2. To permit the patient to tolerate both the oral tube and I.P.P.R. after regaining consciousness he found that phenoperidine and haloperidol were invaluable.
3. By deferring extubation for some hours in this way, the need to perform a tracheostomy could frequently be avoided.
According to REES an addition of 20% nitrous oxide is sufficient, while HOLMDAHL prefers to give 10% nitrous oxide and 1 mg phenoperidin every 3 hours.

Gray pointed out that serious damage to hemopoesis in the bone marrow, which had formerly developed after 3 days when 60% nitrous oxide was given to tetanus patients, was not observed in the Soviet Union when 50% of nitrous oxide was given for up to 3 days. Indications and advantages of respirator treatment after heart operations were discussed by HOLMDAHL.

Yamamura reported on the control of acid-base balance during open heart surgery especially with hypothermia is very important problem. But much controversy exist about the presence of changes in acid-base and their connection during and following hypothermia.
1. How to calculate base excess or deficit during cardiopulmonary bypass with hypothermia?

If the patient is at normal temperature, base excess or deficit is obtained by SIGGAARD-ANDERSEN nomogram by measuring the pCO^2 and pH of blood sample. But if the patient becomes hypothermic, is this nomogram still useful to derive base excess or deficit?

The use of the nomogram is an ideal method of estimating the change in buffering capacity of the blood whatever the temperature of the blood when it is removed from the patient. ANDERSEN says that if it is desired to use this nomogram as a measure of the accumulation of non-volatile acid or base in hypothermic patient, the analysis must be done at 38° C, and not at the actual temperature and also that the base excess value is independent of temperature. Thus, we can calculate base excess or deficit by measuring pCO^2 and pH of blood sample at 38°C. In other words, we can measure base excess or deficit with the same method as in the normothermic patient.

CARSON and others are measuring base deficit (during cardiopulmonary bypass with hypothermia) with this method.

On the other hand, some people do not agree with this method of calculation.

ALEXANDER says that if we want to measure base deficit or excess during hypothermia, the pH and pCO_2 which were measured at 37° C should be corrected to body temperature. The correction of pH is done by using ROSENTHAL's factor and that of pCO_2 is done by using SEVERINGHAUS nomogram. And the values should be referred to a pH-bicarbonate diagram which have also been corrected for body temperature.

According to him, the use of the SIGGAARD-ANDERSEN nomogram will always result in an overestimation of buffer base concentration.

I do not know which is the better method. Anyway with regard to base excess or deficit, data on temperature changes have not been found in the literature. This problem needs further investigation and when we discuss acid base balance, we must say which method we have used.

As far as our study is concerned, we used the former method and we have found that metabolic acidosis occurred during perfusion under hypothermia.

2. What is the optimum acid base value in cardiopulmonary bypass with hypothermia?

Both EDMARK and OSBORN confirmed the desirability of lowering pH during extracorporeal circulation and hypothermia. They lowered pH with hydrochloric acid and observed less cardiac irritability and lower incidence of ventricular fibrillation. In addition, they say that patients controlled in this way have a decreased morbidity and a smooth postoperative course.

CARSON used CO_2 into the pump oxygenator and lowered the pH to the predetermined level. According to him, this technique prevents the occurrence of metabolic acidosis and greatly reduces the myocardial irritability usually associated with hypothermia.

On the other hand Zingg says fluctuation of the pH should be avoided during cardiopulmonary bypass except for a temporary lowering. A temporary lowering of the pH with CO_2 is favorable for defibrillation.

Other people are trying to maintain pH in the region of 7.4 and pCO_2 in the region of 40 mm Hg during hypothermia.

It is very difficult to decide which is better to keep the pH around 7.4 or lower during hypothermia. This problem also needs further investigation.

However respiratory alkalosis is to be avoided. Respiratory alkalosis appears to result in a base deficit which is subsequently revealed as a metabolic acidosis. According to our study, if metabolic acidosis is found before perfusion, it is still present after the perfusion and hypothermia.

3. Which is better to treat metabolic acidosis with sod. bicarbonate or with Tris buffer?

In case of moderate acidosis, sod. bicarbonate is satisfactory. But in case of severe acidosis, the use of sod. bicarbonate may result in a large amount of sodium being given. Furthermore, bicarbonate dose not enter the cells. Whereas Tris buffer enters the cells where it may act as an intracellular buffer. Tris buffer also has an osmotic diuretic action that helps to maintain good urinary output.

Stead reported: It is only fair to say that the incidence of neurological complications, presumably caused by blood sludging, has become so serious a factor that steps are now taken to maintain cerebral perfusion as near normal as possible throughout operation. This implies normal temperature, pCO_2 and adequate extracellular volumes during anaesthesia, and the use of Rheomacrodex in the post-operative period. It seems that only d-tubocurarine is responsible for the maintenance of sleep now!

Rees reported on thoughts on the maintenance of unconsciousness during cardiopulmonary bypass.

In formulating a system of anaesthesia for cardiopulmonary bypass operations, among the problems that require consideration is that of the maintenance of unconsciousness during the actual bypass. There are two principal choices open to the anaesthetic team undertaking this work. On the one hand the technique may involve the administration to the patient or into the oxygenator small quantities of non-volatile agents such as barbiturates or phenothiazine derivatives or analgesic drugs, e.g. pethidine. While this approach will ensure unconsciousness it necessarily reduces the capacity of the heart to perform work at the moment in time when this is most undesirable. Not only has the heart to adjust itself to the alteration of haemodynamics consequent upon the operation but its capacity to do so is affected by the ventriculotomy with the entailed cutting of coronary vessels. A high cardiac output under these conditions may be difficult to achieve.

On the other hand, the anaesthetist may decide to use a relaxant hyperventilation technique, employing nitrous oxide/oxygen as his only anaesthetic agents and by the reduction of the pCO_2 to levels in the low twenties to produce not only unconsciousness but a high degree of "analgesia". If the pCO_2 level can be prevented from rising during bypass, as is certainly possible in paediatrics, then the patient will be unaware of surgery. The depression of cardiac function caused by operation will not be enhanced by drug administration and in the poor risk patient this may be decisive.

The objective of any bypass technique is, however, the provision of a normal cell perfusion particularly the brain cells. The adoption of a particular means for maintaining unconsciousness during bypass cannot be made without appreciation of the effects this may have on tissue perfusion itself. Extreme hyperventilation causes intense vasoconstriction which may lead in cardiac surgery to an inadequate cerebral perfusion. If this technique is employed then a reduction of blood viscosity by the addition of dextrose water to the priming blood is a necessary corollary. If, however, anaesthetic agents, e.g. halothane, phenergan and pethidine, are used and hyperventilation is avoided the dilatory effects of these drugs enable whole blood to be used to prime the oxygenator. Our own preference is for the technique which employs the minimum of toxic drugs.

G. Recent advances in intravenous anaesthetics for ambulatory patients*

Chairman: M. Zindler, Düsseldorf
Members: A. Doenicke, Munich; J. W. Dundee, Belfast; V. Goldman,
London; T. Howells, London; I. A. Illes, Chicago; P. A. Radnay,
New York; H. Sankawa, Los Angeles.

M. Zindler, of Düsseldorf (Germany), was the chairman of the first
panel discussion, dealing with advantages and disadvantages of intravenous
anaesthetics and reaching the conclusion that derivatives of phenoxyacetic
acid are especially suitable for short anaesthesia of out-patients. – Doenicke
of Munich (Germany), Dundee of Belfast (Ireland), Goldman and Howells
(of London), Illes (of Chicago), Radnay (of New York) and Sankawa
(of Los Angeles) reported their favourable experience with the new preparation propanidid and compared it with the short-acting barbiturate methohexital. – The contribution on physico-chemical and pharmacological
properties of several barbiturates and thiobarbiturates established that
there are differences in the potency and duration of action between thiopental, thiobutabarbital and methohexital, depending on the fat solubility of
the substance, the serum concentration and the rate of binding to serum
protein. Protein binding also plays an essential role in the post-anaesthetic
effects. Designating these barbiturates compounds "ultra-short acting
anaesthetics" is misleading and unacceptable. They can only be referred to
as quickly acting anaesthetics. An essential aspect of outpatient anaesthesia
is the post-anaesthetic phase. EEG monitoring has shown that this phase is
marked by sleep curves after the mentioned barbiturates and thiobarbiturates,
sleep spindles impairing the patient's reactivity and "street fitness" occuring
for as long as 12–24 hours post-anaesthetically. – These findings substantiate
interest in propanidid, a new derivative of phenoxyacetate, as a suitable
anaesthetic for out-patients. A discussion of the pharmacology of the compound revealed rapid breakdown (esteratic splitting) in the body into
anaesthetically inactive metabolites as the prominent factor. This splitting
begins during the first blood circulation, and anaesthesia of only 3–4 min

---

* The complete text of this panel has appeared as Supplementum XVII of
the Acta Anaesthesiologica Scandinavica.

duration is achieved. The indications for this short-acting anaesthetic thus emerge immediately. – Anaesthesia can be prolonged by subsequent injection of propanidid or change to another anaesthetic agent. Children between 2–12 years need on average 10 mg/kg (adults 5–8 mg) of propanidid intravenously. A few failures that have been observed were apparently connected with excessive or chronic alcoholism. – When discussing the particular features of propanidid anaesthesia all members of the panel agreed that it begins within 30 sec of the injection. An initial brief phase of hyperventilation is followed by moderate respiratory depression. While the blood pressure falls somewhat during the first minute, the pulse rate temporarily rises. Preanaesthetic values are usually regained within 2–3 min. A few instances of a more marked hypotension that were observed concerned mostly elderly or cachectic patients, and it is recommended to give only half the usual dosage in poor-risk cases. General and local tolerance, too, were discussed and compared with barbiturates. – Psychological testing and EEG monitoring confirmed that phenoxyacetate derivatives have an actually short post-anaesthetic phase, full reactivity being restituted 20–30 min after the anaesthesia. – Consideration of all applying aspects led the panel to the following *conclussion:* The suitability of thiobarbiturates and methohexital for out-patient anaesthesia is limited by a long post-anaesthetic phase, sleep stages appearing for as long as 12–24 hrs after the anaesthesia. The phenoxy-acetate derivatives can be designated genuinely short-acting anaesthetics – particularly on the basis of the rapid restitution of reactivity post-anaesthetically.

H. Hypotension

Chairman: J. E. ECKENHOFF, Philadelphia
Members: S. ELLIS, Philadelphia; G. E. H. ENDERBY, London; W. K. HAMILTON, Iowa City; O. V. S. KOK, Pretoria.

The problems of artificial hypotension were reviewed in this excellent panel discussion which was directed by J. E. ECKENHOFF (Philadelphia).

Relationships of blood pressure, peripheral blood flow and oxygen demand of tissues were illuminated by results of experiments and clinical experiences.

L. HAVERS (Bonn) observed surprisingly little difference regarding the influence on liver function tests between normo- and hypotensive halothane anaesthetics in patients with hepatic cirrhosis as well as patients with normal liver function. Generally, Arfonad is preferred to achieve prolonged hypotension. M. SCHÄDLICH and ERLACH (Charité, Berlin) reported about good experiences with artificial hypotension by intravenous procain drip infusion. Ganglionic blockade is again recommended for the treatment of shock, in in septic shock in combination with Terravenós and high doses of cortisone (up to 800 mg).

It was summarized that artificial hypotension is to be considered a serious procedure which may even be burned by mortality; it has, nevertheless, a place among the anaesthetic techniques of today.

Panel discussions on

I. Neuroleptanalgesia

Chairman: C. R. RITSEMA VAN ECK, Groningen
Members: A. S. BROWN, Edinburgh; G. CORSSEN, Ann Arbor; J. F. CRUL,
Nijmegen; M. GEMPERLE, Geneva; W. F. HENSCHEL, Bremen; M. KEERI-
SZANTO, Montreal; E. NILSSON, Lund; F. F. FOLDES, New York, assistent
by C. V, MORPURGO, Milan.

The chairman indroduces the topic of the panel and announces that due to
the newness of the subject the panel will be more of a symposion on neuroleptanalgesia, than a panel.

The participants will mostly resort to a short exposé of certain aspects of
the neuroleptanalgesia.

Dr. J.F. CRUL starts with the pharmacology, and the results of animal experiments and is followed by Dr. F. F. FOLDES, who adds some clinical experiments in which it is proved that phentanyl is $\pm$ 1000 $\times$ more effective
as an analgesic than meperidine; that droperidol does not effect the respiratory depression of meperidine, but does so in the case of phentanyl; that
narcotic antagonists reverse the action of phentanyl effectively. Dr. M .GEM-
PERLE shows in dog experiments that although oxygen uptake is less, metabolism is so much reduced, that the animal is better oxygenated. Dr. E.
NILSSON accentuates the fact, that with these analgesics (phenoperidin and
phentanyl) one can selectively depress pain perception without depressing
consciousness, a very noteworthy observation. He talked on brain circulation, which seemed to be increased. Dr. W. F. HENSCHEL discussed the
technique mostly in use. Also he commented on a report of Dr. BOGER
and Dr. TORNETTA, Pennsylvania, on liverfunktion, which showed no evidence of liver damage, which was confirmed by Dr. M. KEERI-SZANTO, who
also spoke on the use in geriatric patients and could confirm the observations of the others on the low toxicity of the drugs and their stabilizing
effect on circulation.

Dr. A. S. BROWN and Dr. J. F. CRUL commented on the use in short and
diagnostic procedures and the side-actions (pyramidal and rigidity). Dr. C.
V. MORPURGO and Dr. W. F. HENSCHEL gave some data of the use in
children, an aspect that is still in development. Dr. G. CORSSEN recommended the use of neuroleptanalgesia in open heart surgery.

J. Problems of anaesthetics in developing regions

Chairman: Sir Robert R. Macintosh, Oxford
Members: R. Ghose, Addis Abeba; Q. J. Gomez, Manila; R. A. Gordon, Toronto; R. A. Hingson, Cleveland; K. A. Oduro, Accra; G. S. W. Organe, London; K. F. Stephens, London; I. Wakai, Nagoya.

This panel discussion was directed by Sir Robert Macintosh (Oxford). Sir Robert Macintosh is familiar with the conditions in all continents by own experience, he has favorably influenced the development of anaesthesia in many countries around the world by travels and lectures. In the course of the discussion it was emphasized several times that there is little advantage in having complicated machines for inhalation anaesthesia in remote places because of difficulties and expense of service and replacement of oxygen- and nitrous oxide cylinders. It was reported about good experiences with the Epstein-Macintosh-Oxford (EMO) apparatus for ether-air-anaesthesia; the EMO apparatus allows also artificial respiration.

In the majority of the hospitals in underdeveloped countries anaesthetics are given by non-anaesthetists, often by nurses. Postgraduate training is difficult because the physician cannot afford to be absent from his hospital for any length of time to participate in a training course of a university. If younger fellows are sent to the United States for training they often prefer working-and living conditions there and do not return to their native countries. This is the reason why instructors should be sent to the hospitals of underdeveloped countries to advance anaesthesia there.